Student Lab Manual for

Wilson: Health Assessment for Nursing Practice

Sixth Edition

Susan Fickertt Wilson, PhD, RN

Emeritus Associate Professor
Harris College of Nursing and Health Sciences
Texas Christian University
Fort Worth, Texas

Jean Foret Giddens, PhD, RN, FAAN

Dean and Professor
Yingling Chair of Nursing
School of Nursing
Virginia Commonwealth University
Richmond, Virginia

Reviewer:

Bobbie Dixon, MSN, RN

Assistant Professor
College of Nursing
University of Mary Hardin-Baylor
Belton, Texas

ELSEVIER

ELSEVIER

3251 Riverport Lane
St. Louis, Missouri 63043

*Student Laboratory Manual for Health Assessment for
Nursing Practice*, Sixth Edition

ISBN: 978-0-323-37783-6

Notices

Knowledge and best practice in this field are constantly changing. As new research and experience broaden our understanding, changes in research methods, professional practices, or medical treatment may become necessary.

Practitioners and researchers must always rely on their own experience and knowledge in evaluating and using any information, methods, compounds, or experiments described herein. In using such information or methods they should be mindful of their own safety and the safety of others, including parties for whom they have a professional responsibility.

With respect to any drug or pharmaceutical products identified, readers are advised to check the most current information provided (i) on procedures featured or (ii) by the manufacturer of each product to be administered, to verify the recommended dose or formula, the method and duration of administration, and contraindications. It is the responsibility of practitioners, relying on their own experience and knowledge of their patients, to make diagnoses, to determine dosages and the best treatment for each individual patient, and to take all appropriate safety precautions.

To the fullest extent of the law, neither the Publisher nor the authors, contributors, or editors assume any liability for any injury and/or damage to persons or property as a matter of products liability, negligence or otherwise, or from any use or operation of any methods, products, instructions, or ideas contained in the material herein.

ISBN: 978-0-323-37783-6

Content Strategist: Lee Henderson
Content Development Specialist: Laura Goodrich
Publishing Services Manager: Hemamalini Rajendrababu
Project Manager: Nadhiya Sekar
Cover Designer: Muthukumaran Thangaraj

Printed in the United States of America

Last digit is the print number: 9 8 7 6 5 4 3 2 1

Working together
to grow libraries in
developing countries

www.elsevier.com • www.bookaid.org

Contents

CHAPTER 1   Importance of Health Assessment

No laboratory activities are required for the content in this chapter.

CHAPTER 2 Obtaining a Health History

With your lab partner assuming the role of a patient, conduct a comprehensive history. Your "student patient" may role-play a person with particular related symptoms and history.

HISTORY

BIOGRAPHIC DATA

Date	Name		Gender M F
Date of birth	Age	Race	Marital status S M D W	Occupation

REASON FOR SEEKING HEALTH CARE (Presenting problem)

HISTORY OF PRESENT ILLNESS

Symptom Analysis of Presenting Problem (Onset, Location, Duration, Characteristics, Aggravating and Alleviating factors, Related symptoms, Treatment, Severity)

Present Health Status (current health conditions/chronic illnesses)

Current Medications: (Include prescription, over-the-counter, herbs, and vitamins)
(Document if no medications are taken)

Name of Drug	Dosage/Frequency	Last Dose Taken	Reason for Taking

Current Medical Treatments (e.g., breathing treatments, dialysis, wound dressing):
(Document if no medical treatments are used)

Allergies to Medication/Foods/Medical Products/Other (e.g., latex, contrast, tape)
(Document if there are no allergies)

Allergic To	Reaction

PAST HEALTH HISTORY

Childhood Illnesses (Check all that apply):

Measles ❑	Mumps ❑	Rubella ❑	Chickenpox ❑
Pertussis ❑	Influenza ❑	Ear infections ❑	Throat infections ❑
Other (describe) ❑			

List previous medical conditions, surgeries, hospitalizations, or injuries. (Document if none apply)

Name and Type	Date	Residual Problems

Immunization	Date/s	Immunization	Date/s
Diphtheria, tetanus, acellular pertussis (DTaP)		*Haemophilus influenzae* type b (Hib)	
Hepatitis A		Hepatitis B	
Human papillomavirus (HPV)		Inactivated poliomyelitis (IPV)	
Influenza vaccine		Measles, mumps, rubella (MMR)	
Meningococcal conjugate vaccine (MCV)		Pneumococcal conjugate (PCV13)	
Pneumococcal polysaccharide (PPSV23)		Rotavirus	
Tetanus (Td)		Varicella	
Other		Other	

Last Examination	Date	Outcome
Last Physical		
Last Vision		
Last Dental		
Other (describe)		
Women Only		
Last Menstrual Period (LMP)		
Last Pregnancy		Gravida (number of pregnancies) _____ Para (number of births) _____ Abortion/miscarriage _____
Last Pap Smear		
Last Mammogram		

Family History (Indicate age and current health. If deceased, indicate age and cause of death.)

Person	Age	Current Health	Person	Age	Current Health
Mother			Father		
Sister			Brother		
Sister			Brother		
Daughter			Son		
Daughter			Son		

Draw a genogram for your lab partner's family history.

PERSONAL AND PSYCHOSOCIAL HISTORY

Personal Status (feelings about self, cultural/religious affiliations and practices, education / work satisfaction, hobbies and interests)

Family and Social Relationships (significant others, individuals in home, role within family)

Diet / Nutrition (appetite, typical food and fluid intake, dietary restrictions, use of dietary supplements)

Functional Ability (indicate ability to independently perform the following self-care activities[†])

Dressing ❑   Toileting ❑   Bathing ❑   Eating ❑

Ambulating ❑   Shopping ❑   Cooking ❑   Housekeeping ❑

[†]If unable to perform independently, describe.

Mental Health (stress, anxiety, depression, irritability, personal coping strategies)

Tobacco, Alcohol, and Illicit Drug Use

Tobacco use:	Y ❑	N ❑	Packs per day:	
Alcohol intake:	Y ❑	N ❑	Drinks per day:	
Illicit drug use:	Y ❑	N ❑	Describe:	

Health Promotion Practices   **Describe**

Exercise (type/frequency):	
Stress management:	
Sleep habits:	
Self-examination (type/frequency):	
Use of seat belts:	
Other:	

Environment (Include living and work environment)

Safety devices: (e.g., smoke alarms)	
Potential hazards:	
Within home	
Within neighborhood	

REVIEW OF SYSTEMS (Check all that apply and comment below; document if no symptoms reported)

General Symptoms			
Pain ❑	Fatigue ❑	Weakness ❑	Fever ❑
Problems sleeping ❑	Unexplained changes in weight ❑		
Comments:			

Integumentary System			
Skin lesions ❑	Excessive dryness ❑	Change in a mole ❑	Changes in skin color, texture ❑
Sore that does not heal ❑	Rashes ❑	Itching ❑	Frequent bruising ❑
Changes in amount, texture, distribution of hair ❑	Changes in texture, color of nails ❑	Use of sunscreen ❑	
Comments:			

Head			
Headaches ❑	Head injury ❑	Dizziness ❑	Fainting spells ❑
Use of protective head gear ❑			
Comments:			

Eyes			
Change in vision ❑	Discharge ❑	Excessive tearing ❑	Eye pain ❑
Sensitivity to light ❑	Flashing lights ❑	Halos around lights ❑	Difficulty reading ❑
Blurred vision ❑	Do you wear corrective lenses? ❑	If yes: Eyeglasses ❑	Contact lenses ❑
Comments:			

Ears			
Ear pain ❑	Discharge ❑	Recurrent infections ❑	Excessive earwax ❑
Changes in hearing ❑	Ringing in ears ❑	Sensitivity to noises ❑	Use of hearing device ❑
Protect ears from excessively loud noises ❑			
Comments:			

Nose, Nasopharynx, Sinuses			
Nasal discharge ❑	Frequent nosebleeds ❑	Sneezing ❑	Nasal obstruction ❑
Sinus pain ❑	Postnasal drip ❑	Change in smell ❑	Snoring ❑
Comments:			

Mouth/Oropharynx			
Sore throat ❑	Sore in mouth ❑	Bleeding gums ❑	Change in taste ❑
Trouble chewing ❑	Trouble swallowing ❑	Dental prosthesis ❑	Change in voice ❑
Oral hygiene practice (frequency of brushing/ flossing) ❑			
Comments:			

Neck

Lymph node enlargement ❑	Swelling or mass in neck ❑	Neck pain ❑	Neck stiffness ❑
Comments:			

Breasts

Pain ❑	Swelling ❑	Lumps or masses ❑	Change in appearance ❑
Nipple discharge ❑			
Comments:			

Respiratory System

Cough ❑	Shortness of breath (dyspnea) ❑	Frequent colds ❑	Pain with breathing ❑
Wheezing ❑	Coughing up blood (hemoptysis) ❑	Night sweats ❑	Exposure to smoke ❑
Handwashing ❑	Influenza vaccine ❑	Smoking cessation ❑	
Comments:			

Cardiovascular System

Chest pain ❑	Palpitations ❑	Shortness of breath (dyspnea) ❑	Dyspnea during sleep ❑
Edema ❑	Coldness to extremities ❑	Discoloration ❑	Varicose veins ❑
Leg pain with activity ❑	Paresthesia ❑	Limit salt and fat intake ❑	Cholesterol screening ❑
Blood pressure screening ❑	Exercise/activity ❑		
Comments:			

Gastrointestinal System

Pain ❑	Heartburn ❑	Nausea/vomiting ❑	Vomiting blood ❑
Jaundice ❑	Change in appetite ❑	Diarrhea ❑	Constipation ❑
Blood in stools ❑	Hemorrhoids ❑	Change in bowel habits ❑	Dietary analysis ❑
Colon cancer screening ❑			
Comments:			

Urinary System

Hesitancy ❑	Frequency ❑	Urgency ❑	Change in urine stream ❑
Excessive urination at night ❑	Pain with urination ❑	Flank pain ❑	Blood in urine ❑
Incontinence ❑	Excessive urination ❑	Decreased urination ❑	

Comments:

Reproductive System

Male:	Lesions ❑	Pain ❑	Masses ❑	Penile discharge ❑
	Hernia ❑			
Female:	Lesions ❑	Pain ❑	Vaginal discharge ❑	Absent menses ❑
	Painful menses ❑	Irregular menses ❑		

Sexual Activity

Are you currently involved in a sexual relationship(s)?	❑ No ❑ Yes, what is the nature of the relationship(s)?
Number of sexual partners in last 3 months?	
Do you protect yourself from sexually transmitted diseases (STDs)?	❑ No ❑ Yes, what method is used?
Do you use birth control?	❑ No ❑ Yes, what method is used?

Problems with sexual activity

Painful intercourse ❑	Change in sex drive ❑	Infertility ❑	Impotence ❑	

Comments:

Musculoskeletal System

Muscle pain ❑	Muscle weakness ❑	Joint swelling ❑	Joint pain ❑
Joint stiffness ❑	Deformity/crepitus ❑	Limitations in range of motion ❑	Back pain ❑
Use of body mechanics ❑	Osteoporosis screening ❑		

Comments:

Neurologic System			
Pain ❑	Seizures ❑	Fainting ❑	Changes in cognition ❑
Changes in memory ❑	Problems with coordination ❑	Tremor ❑	Spasms ❑
Changes in sensation ❑	Disorientation ❑		
Comments:			

CLINICAL REASONING

1. Organize or cluster your findings for this patient by body system or concepts.

2. Analyze data collected. (Which data deviate from expected findings? Which additional data are needed?)

3. Using the analysis above, determine nursing diagnoses for this patient.

CHAPTER 3 Techniques and Equipment for Physical Assessment

With a lab partner, practice these examination techniques.

Examination Techniques	Document Findings
Inspection Inspect the skin on the forearm of your lab partner. What is the overall color? Do you see any variations in color or texture? Note the hair on the arm—amount, color, patterns. Do you see a lesion (scar, mole) on the forearm? If so, where is it located and what size is it?	Color: Hair color/distribution: Lesions:

Palpation
With your lab partner, practice light palpation with your fingertips and deep palpation with your hands. In the column to the right, indicate the type of palpation appropriate for the example given.
 	
Touch the skin of your lab partner. Note the temperature, moisture, and skin texture. Document your palpation findings at the right.
	Palpate a radial pulse.
	  deep light
	
	Palpate the texture of skin.
	  deep light
	
	Palpate the abdomen.
	  deep light
	
	Palpate tenderness over a muscle.
	  deep light
	
	Skin Palpation
	  Temperature:
	
	  Moisture:
	
	  Texture:

Examination Techniques	Document Findings
Percussion Practice indirect finger percussion using the surface of the following three objects: an empty cardboard box, a table surface, and a liquid-filled plastic container. • Can you hear percussion tones? • Can you hear differences in the tones of the various objects?	Empty cardboard box: Table surface: Liquid-filled plastic container:
Examination Techniques Practice indirect finger percussion with your lab partner. Percuss over the following places: abdomen over the stomach; abdomen over the liver; chest over the lung field; and chest over the sternum. • Can you hear percussion tones? • Can you hear differences in tones as you percuss the different areas?	Abdomen-stomach: Abdomen-liver: Chest-lung: Chest-sternum:

Examination Techniques	Document Findings	Yes	No
Auscultation With your lab partner, listen through your stethoscope and attempt to hear sounds at the following locations: abdomen, carotid artery, lungs, heart, brachial artery. Indicate "Y" or "N" whether you can hear sounds.	Abdomen	❏	❏
	Carotid artery	❏	❏
	Lungs	❏	❏
	Heart	❏	❏
	Brachial artery	❏	❏

EQUIPMENT

With a lab partner, complete the following activities using the equipment available in your lab.

Thermometers

Electronic thermometer:

• Put a disposable sheath over the probe. What is the temperature? _____

• What temperature unit is the electronic thermometer calibrated in?

Fahrenheit ❏   Celsius ❏   Both ❏

Tympanic thermometer:

- Put a disposable sheath over the probe. What is the temperature? _____

- What temperature unit is the electronic thermometer calibrated in?

    Fahrenheit ❑   Celsius ❑   Both ❑

Temporal artery thermometer:

- Depress the scan button on the thermometer and slide across one side of the lab partner's forehead to behind the ear. What is the temperature? _____

- What temperature unit is the electronic thermometer calibrated in?

    Fahrenheit ❑   Celsius ❑   Both ❑

Stethoscope

- Identify the following parts of your stethoscope: earpiece, tubing, head (bell and diaphragm).

- If your stethoscope has a two-sided head, turn it to the bell and then to the diaphragm. How can you tell which side is engaged?

- Place the earpieces in your ears, pointing forward. Gently rub or tap the head of the stethoscope to elicit sound.

Sphygmomanometer/Cuffs

- Practice placing and removing a cuff on your lab partner's arm.

- Compare various sizes of cuffs. Practice steps involved in determining a correct fit on your lab partner.

- Holding the cuff tightly wrapped in your hand, practice inflating the cuff with the inflation bulb, then slowly deflate the cuff using the control knob next to the inflation bulb.

- If your lab has one, examine an electronic blood pressure device. How does the procedure for placing a cuff differ compared with the manual BP cuffs?

- Determine how to turn the device on and off. Identify the display for blood pressure measurement. What other information is displayed?

Doppler

- If available, read the instructions that accompany the Doppler.

- Turn the Doppler on and listen to the vascular tones over the radial or brachial artery of your lab partner. What sounds do you hear over the vessel?

Pulse Oximeter

- If available, review the instructions for using the pulse oximeter.

- Turn on the device, place the probe on the finger of your lab partner, and record the oxygen saturation of arterial blood (SaO_2).

  Level = _____%

- What does this mean?

Ophthalmoscope

- Learn how to put on and take off the head of the ophthalmoscope.

- What is the power source for your instrument?

- Turn on the power switch to your instrument. Shine the light from the instrument against your hand. Turn the aperture dial and observe the various settings: large light, small light, red-free filter, slit light, and grid light. As you shine these on your hand, identify each setting.

- Locate the lens selector dial. Turn the lens and observe the red and black numbers.

- Look through the eyepiece at your hand (or another object) and slowly turn the lens selector dial. Become familiar with adjusting the magnification while looking through the eyepiece.

Otoscope

- Learn how to put on and take off the head of the otoscope.

- What is the power source for your instrument?

- Compare adult and pediatric speculums (black, cone-shaped pieces).

- Place a speculum on the head of the otoscope.

- Turn on the power switch to your instrument. Shine the light from the instrument against your hand.

- Look through the lens at your hand or another small object.

Tuning Fork

- Identify the type or types of tuning forks available in your lab.

- Strike the tuning fork against the palm of your hand. Are you able to hear and feel vibrations?

Goniometer

- Inspect the goniometer. What is the calibration for measurement?

- Set the goniometer at the following angles: 90°, 60°, 110°, 45°, 10°, 20°

- Ask your lab partner to partially flex his or her elbow. Attempt to measure the angle with the goniometer.

Skin-Fold Calipers

- Read the instructions that come with the calipers, if available.

- Inspect the calipers. What are the calibrations for measurement?

- Manipulate the calipers. Measure the thickness of a small book, a pen or pencil, and a cell phone.

  Book _____ Pen/pencil _____ Cell phone _____

Ruler and Tape Measure

- Note the units of measurement on your ruler: Tape measure:

- Measure the following spots with your ruler. Write your measurements in the space provided.

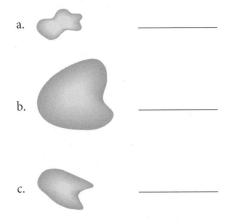

  a. _____

  b. _____

  c. _____

- Measure the circumference of your lab partner's left wrist and his or her left forearm, 4 inches below the elbow.

  Record your measurements.   Left wrist _____   Left forearm _____

CHAPTER 4 General Inspection and Measurement of Vital Signs

GENERAL INSPECTION

In the space to the right, document a general inspection of your lab partner. Use the information at the left for help.

Examination Techniques	Findings (document findings below)
Physical Appearance / Hygiene General appearance: Does patient appear healthy? Is appearance consistent with stated age? Note general color of skin and general hygiene. Is patient well groomed?	**Physical Appearance / Hygiene**
Body Structure and Position Observe general stature. Does the patient appear well nourished? Is the body symmetric? Note the position or posture. Is it comfortable and relaxed? Are there any obvious deformities? Is the patient having trouble breathing?	**Body Structure**
Body Movement Observe the patient's movement. Does the patient walk with ease? Is the gait balanced and smooth with symmetric movement of extremities? Do there appear to be any limitations to range of motion? Are there any involuntary movements?	**Body Movement**
Emotional/Mental Status and Behavior Is the patient alert? Does the patient maintain eye contact? Does the patient converse appropriately? Are facial expressions and body language appropriate for the conversation? Is the dress appropriate for the weather? Is the behavior appropriate?	**Emotional/Mental Status and Behavior**

MEASUREMENT OF VITAL SIGNS

With a lab partner, complete the following activities using the equipment available in your lab.

PERFORM hand hygiene.

Temperature

Measure your lab partner's temperature using different routes. Use a variety of thermometers if your lab has different ones available. Compare the results.

Temperature	Reading (circle scale)
Oral	F C
Axillary	F C
Tympanic	F C
Temporal artery	F C

Heart Rate

Measure your lab partner's heart rate by taking a pulse. Take the pulse in the three locations indicated below. Count the pulse for 15 seconds and multiply by 4, or count the pulse for 30 seconds and multiply by 2. Do you get the same pulse rate in each location? Document the rate and circle the rhythm.

	Brachial		Radial		Carotid	
	15 sec × 4	30 sec × 2	15 sec × 4	30 sec × 2	15 sec × 4	30 sec × 2

Heart Rate	Rate
	
	Rhythm
	
	  Regular
	
	  Regularly
	    irregular
	
	  Irregularly
	    irregular
			Rate
			
			Rhythm
			
			  Regular
			
			  Regularly
			    irregular
			
			  Irregularly
			    irregular
					Rate
					
					Rhythm
					
					  Regular
					
					  Regularly
					    irregular
					
					  Irregularly
					    irregular	

Respiratory Rate

Count the respiratory rate of your lab partner in both a sitting and supine position. Count the breaths for 15 seconds and multiply by 4, or count for 30 seconds and multiply by 2.

	Sitting		Supine	
	15 sec × 4	30 sec × 2	15 sec × 4	30 sec × 2
Respirations	Rate Quality Depth	Rate	Rate Quality Depth	Rate

- Which position is easier to count respirations? (Indicate sitting or supine.)

Blood Pressure

While your lab partner is in both a supine and sitting position, take a blood pressure reading in both arms using a manual blood pressure device. Record your findings below.

	Sitting		Supine	
	Right Arm	**Left Arm**	**Right Arm**	**Left Arm**
Blood pressure				

- If your lab has one, take your lab partner's blood pressure using an electronic blood pressure device.

- Are the readings using the electronic device different than your manual readings? Are the blood pressures different with position changes or between the two arms? If a difference is noted, what might account for this difference?

Height/Weight

- Measure your lab partner's height in both inches and centimeters: _____ in _____ cm

- Measure your lab partner's weight in both pounds and kilograms: _____ lbs _____ kg

- Use Table 8-4 in Chapter 8 to determine your lab partner's body mass index (BMI): _____

CHAPTER 5 Cultural Assessment

With your lab partner assuming the role of a patient, conduct a cultural assessment. Your "student patient" may role-play a person with particular related symptoms and history.

HISTORY

BIOGRAPHIC DATA

Date	Name	Gender M F
Date of birth	Age	Race	Marital status S M D W	Occupation

PERSONAL AND PSYCHOSOCIAL HISTORY

Introductory Questions

- Where were you born?

- With what particular cultural group (or groups) do you identify?

- Which cultural practices are important to you?

Primary Language and Method of Communication

- Which language is usually spoken in your home?

- How well do you speak, read, and write English?

- In which language do you think?

- Will you need the services of a translator during the time you are in this health care facility?

- Are there any special rituals of communication in your family? (For example, is there someone to whom questions should be directed?) Tell me about these.

- Are there any unique customs in your culture that influence the way you speak to someone or the way you behave toward him or her? Tell me about these customs.

- How do you show respect for others?

Personal Beliefs About Health and Illness

- Do you believe that you have control over your health? If not, what or whom do you believe controls it?

- Name some practices or rituals that you believe will improve your health.

- Do you use or have you used any alternative healing methods such as acupuncture, acupressure, ayurvedic medicine, healing touch, or herbal products? If so, how effective were these methods?

- Whom do you consult when you are ill?

- Which specific practices or rituals do you believe should be used to treat your health problem?

- Who makes the health decisions in your family?

- Which health topics do you feel uncomfortable talking about?

- Which examination procedures do you find embarrassing?

- What can the members of the health care team do to help you stay healthy (or become healthy again)?

Beliefs About a Current Health Problem (Sickness)

- What do you call this sickness?

- What do you think caused the sickness?

- Why do you think it started when it did?

- What do you think the sickness does? How does it work?

- How bad is your sickness?

- What kind of treatment do you think you should receive?

- What are the most important results you hope to achieve from this treatment?

- What do you fear most about this sickness?

- What problems has your sickness caused for you?

Religious or Spiritual Influences

- If time or the situation only permits asking one question, ask, "Do you have any spiritual needs or concerns related to your health?"

- Do you have a formal religious affiliation? Please describe it.

- In what ways is your spirituality or religion meaningful to you?

- How is your spirituality or religion important to you in your daily life?

- What practices do you perform as a part of your daily religious and spiritual life (e.g., meditation, prayer, Bible reading)?

- How do your beliefs affect your health practices?

- How does your faith help you cope with illness?

- Are there any specific aspects of medical care that your religion discourages or forbids?

- Are there any religious or spiritual practices or rituals you would like to have available while you are in the hospital?

- What part of your religion or spirituality would you like the nurses to consider as they care for you?

- What knowledge or understanding would strengthen your relationship with the nurses?

Roles in the Family

- Who makes the decisions in your family?

- What is the composition of your family? How many generations or family members live in your household?

- What is the role of children in the family?

- Do you or the other members of your family have any special beliefs and practices about conception, pregnancy, childbirth, lactation, and childrearing?

Special Dietary Practices

- What is the main type of food eaten in your home?

- Are there any foods that are forbidden by your culture or foods that are a cultural requirement? If so, what are they?

- Who in your family is responsible for food preparation?

- How is the food in your culture prepared?

- Are there any specific beliefs or preferences about food, such as those thought to cause or cure illness?

CLINICAL REASONING

1. Organize or cluster your findings for this patient.

2. Based on this cultural assessment, what needs does this person have at this time?

CHAPTER 6   Pain Assessment

With your lab partner assuming the role of a patient, conduct a focused history and examination. Your "student patient" may role-play a person with acute or chronic pain.

HISTORY

BIOGRAPHIC DATA

Date	Name		Gender M F
Date of birth	Age	Race	Marital status S M D W	Occupation

PRESENTING PROBLEM/PROBLEM-BASED HISTORY (These parts of the history are the same when discussing the symptom of pain.)

HISTORY OF PRESENT ILLNESS

Symptom Analysis

- Onset (When does pain occur, onset sudden or gradual, what is cause of pain?)

- Location (Where do you feel the pain?)

- Duration (How long does the pain last?)

- Characteristics (What does the pain feel like?)

- Aggravating factors (What makes the pain worse?)

- Alleviating factors (What make the pain better?)

- Related symptoms (What are other symptoms that you experience during the pain?)

- Treatment (What have you done to relieve the pain? How effective was the treatment?)

- Severity (How would you describe the intensity, strength, or severity of the pain? How severe do you allow your pain to become before you take medication to relieve it?)

Response to Pain

- Does the pain have a particular meaning for you? What is it?

- What has been your past experience with pain and pain relief?

- Do you have any concern about taking medications for pain relief?

- How has pain affected your quality of life? How has it altered your life?

EXAMINATION

Examination Technique	Findings (document findings below)
Routine Techniques	
▶ PERFORM hand hygiene.	
▶ OBSERVE the patient for facial expressions and behavior to relieve pain.	
▶ LISTEN for sounds the patient makes.	
▶ MEASURE blood pressure and PALPATE pulse.	
▶ ASSESS respiratory rate and pattern.	
▶ INSPECT the site of pain for appearance.	
▶ PALPATE the site of pain for tenderness.	

▶ Routine techniques

CLINICAL REASONING

1. Organize or cluster your findings for this patient by body system or concepts.

2. Analyze data collected. (Which data deviate from expected findings? Which additional data are needed?)

3. Using the analysis above, determine nursing diagnoses for this patient.

CHAPTER 7 Mental Health Assessment

For this lab activity, take a history on your lab partner, focusing on a mental health problem. Become familiar with the various screening tools by conducting them on your lab partner.

HISTORY

BIOGRAPHIC DATA

Date	Name				Gender M F
Date of birth	Age	Race		Marital status S M D W	Occupation

PRESENTING PROBLEM (Check all that apply):

Depression ❑   Anxiety ❑   Altered mental status ❑

Alcohol abuse ❑   Drug abuse ❑   Interpersonal violence ❑

Other ❑ _____

PRESENT HEALTH STATUS (chronic conditions and medications, dose, and frequency)

PAST HEALTH HISTORY (behaviors indicating mental health problem, describe your experiences; surgeries, hospitalizations, and accidents/injuries)

FAMILY HISTORY (relatives with mental health problems, any violence in the home)

PERSONAL AND PSYCHOSOCIAL HISTORY

Self-concept: (How have you been feeling about yourself? Do you consider your present feelings to be a problem in your daily life at home or at work or school?)

Interpersonal relationships: (How satisfied are you with your interpersonal relationships?)

Have you been physically injured by someone in your home in the last year? Do you feel safe in your current relationship with your partner?

In the last year, how often did anyone:
- Hurt you physically?

- Insult or talk down to you?

- Threaten you with physical harm?

- Scream or curse at you?

Stressors: (What are the major stressors in your life now? How do you deal with stress? Are these methods of stress relief currently effective for you?)

Anger: (How do you react when you are angry? What happens when you and your partner fight or disagree?)

Alcohol use: (How often do you drink alcohol?)

Illicit drug use: (Do you ever use recreational drugs? Describe your drug use.)

CAGE _____ points (This tool is available at www.addictionsandrecovery.org/addiction-self-test.htm.)

Interpretation of the score: When might you use this?

AUDIT _____ points (See Table 7-2)

Interpretation of the score: When might you use this tool?

HEALTH PROMOTION AND PROTECTION

1. Recommend health promotional activities for this patient.

2. Identify risk factors for this patient.

EXAMINATION

Examination Technique	Findings (document findings below)
Routine Techniques	
▶ PERFORM hand hygiene.	
▶ OBSERVE the patient's gait, posture, and movement.	
▶ NOTICE level of consciousness and affect.	
▶ OBSERVE for appropriate dress and hygiene.	
▶ NOTICE facial expression, voice tone, and flow and rate of speech.	
▶ OBSERVE for perspiration and muscle tension.	
▶ MEASURE blood pressure.	
▶ PALPATE the radial pulse for rate.	
▶ COUNT the respiratory rate and OBSERVE breathing pattern.	
▶ OBSERVE eye movements.	
▶ MEASURE pupil size.	

Examination Technique	Findings (document findings below)
Techniques for Special Circumstances	
* ASSESS mental status[†] by determining: • Orientation • Memory • Calculation ability • Communication skills • Judgment • Abstract reasoning _____ [†]Altered mental status exam is found in problem-based history.	

► Routine techniques
* Special circumstances

CLINICAL REASONING

1. Organize or cluster your findings for this patient.

2. Analyze data collected. (Which data deviate from expected findings? Which additional data are needed?)

3. Determine nursing diagnoses for this patient.

CLINICAL REASONING

1. Organize or cluster your findings for this patient by body system or concepts.

2. Analyze data collected (Which data deviate from expected findings? Which additional data are needed?)

3. Determine nursing diagnoses for this patient.

CHAPTER 8   Nutritional Assessment

With your lab partner assuming the role of a patient, conduct a focused history and examination. Your "student patient" may role-play a person with a particular nutrition-related symptom.

HISTORY

BIOGRAPHIC DATA

Date	Name				Gender M F
Date of birth	Age	Race		Marital status S M D W	Occupation

PRESENTING PROBLEM (Check all that apply):

Weight loss ❑   Weight gain ❑   Difficulty chewing/swallowing ❑   Loss of appetite ❑

Nausea ❑   Other ❑ _____

HISTORY OF PRESENT ILLNESS

Symptom Analysis of Presenting Problem (Onset, Location, Duration, Characteristics, Aggravating and Alleviating factors, Related symptoms, Treatment, Severity)

Present Health Status (chronic illnesses; medications, dose, and frequency; vitamins or dietary supplements; unexplained changes in weight)

Past Health History (concerns relating to weight or problems eating, surgeries for weight loss)

Family History: (nutrition-related problems such as obesity or diabetes mellitus, eating disorder)

Personal and Psychosocial History: (activity level/exercise pattern; dietary restrictions or food allergies; problems obtaining, preparing, or eating food; use of alcohol or street drugs)

Assess Dietary Intake (usual dietary intake)

HEALTH PROMOTION AND PROTECTION

1. Recommend health promotion activities for this patient.

2. Identify risk factors for this patient.

EXAMINATION

Examination Technique	Findings (document findings below)
Routine Techniques	
▶ PERFORM hand hygiene.	
▶ MEASURE height and weight.	Height:
	Weight:
▶ RECORD body mass index using Table 8-4.	BMI:

Examination Technique	Findings (document findings below)
▶ ASSESS general appearance and level of orientation.	
▶ INSPECT skin for surface characteristics, hydration, and lesions.	
▶ INSPECT hair and nails for appearance and texture.	
▶ INSPECT eyes for surface characteristics.	
▶ INSPECT the oral cavity for dentition and intact mucous membranes.	
▶ INSPECT and PALPATE the extremities for shape, size, coordinated movement, and sensation.	
Techniques for Special Circumstances	
✳ CALCULATE desirable body weight (DBW).	
✳ CALCULATE percent change in weight.	
✳ CALCULATE waist-to-hip ratio.	
✳ ESTIMATE body fat by measuring triceps skin fold.	
✳ ASSESS nutritional status by reviewing laboratory tests.	

▶   Routine techniques
✳   Special circumstances

CHAPTER 9 Skin, Hair, and Nails

With your lab partner assuming the role of a patient, conduct a focused history and examination. Your "student patient" may role-play a person with a particular symptom involving the skin, hair, or nails.

HISTORY

BIOGRAPHIC DATA

Date	Name		Gender M F
Date of birth	Age	Race	Marital status S M D W	Occupation

PRESENTING PROBLEM (Check all that apply)

Pruritus ❑   Rash ❑   Pain of skin ❑   Lesion ❑

Changes in mole ❑   Change in skin color ❑   Change in skin texture ❑   Wounds ❑

Changes in hair ❑   Changes in nails ❑   Other ❑ _____

HISTORY OF PRESENT ILLNESS

Symptom Analysis of Presenting Problem (Onset, Location, Duration, Characteristics, Aggravating and Alleviating factors, Related symptoms, Treatment, Severity)

Present Health Status (chronic diseases; medications, dose, and frequency; changes in skin; exposure to chemicals)

Past Health History (diseases or infections of skin or nails, surgeries, accidents)

Family History (skin-related problems such as skin cancer or autoimmune-related disorders)

Personal and Psychosocial History (skin hygiene, health promotion activities: use of sunscreen, skin self-examination, frequency of nail care)

HEALTH PROMOTION AND PROTECTION

1. Recommend health promotion activities for this patient.

2. Identify risk factors for this patient.

EXAMINATION

Examination Technique	Findings (document findings below)
Routine Techniques	
▶ PERFORM hand hygiene.	
Skin ▶ INSPECT the skin for general color.	*Skin*
▶ INSPECT the skin for localized variations in skin color.	
▶ PALPATE the skin for texture, temperature, moisture, mobility, turgor, and thickness.	

Examination Technique	Findings (document findings below)
Hair ▶ INSPECT and PALPATE the scalp and hair for surface characteristics, hair distribution, texture, quantity, and color. ▶ INSPECT facial and body hair for distribution, quantity, and texture.	*Hair*
Nails ▶ INSPECT and PALPATE the nails for shape, contour, consistency, color, thickness, and cleanliness.	*Nails*
Techniques for Special Circumstances	

Skin
✳ INSPECT and PALPATE skin lesions.
  • Primary lesions
 	
  • Secondary lesions
 	
  • Vascular lesions
	Skin

▶   Routine techniques
✳   Special circumstances

CLINICAL REASONING

1. Organize or cluster your findings for this patient by body system or concepts.

2. Analyze data collected. (Which data deviate from expected findings? Which additional data are needed?)

3. Determine nursing diagnoses for this patient.

CHAPTER 10 Head, Eyes, Ears, Nose, and Throat

With your lab partner assuming the role of a patient, conduct a focused history and examination. Your "student patient" may role-play a person with a particular symptom involving the head, eyes, ears, nose, and throat

HISTORY

BIOGRAPHIC DATA

Date	Name				Gender M F
Date of birth	Age	Race		Marital status S M D W	Occupation

PRESENTING PROBLEM (CHECK ALL THAT APPLY):

Head: Headaches ❏   Dizziness or vertigo ❏   Other ❏

Eyes: Difficulty with vision ❏   Other ❏

Ears: Hearing loss ❏   Ringing in ears ❏   Earache ❏   Other ❏

Nose: Nasal drainage ❏   Nosebleeds ❏   Other ❏

Mouth/Throat: Sore throat ❏   Mouth lesion ❏   Other ❏

HISTORY OF PRESENT ILLNESS

Symptom Analysis of Presenting Problem (Onset, Location, Duration, Characteristics, Aggravating and Alleviating factors, Related symptoms, Treatment, Severity)

Present Health Status (changes to head, eyes, ears, nose, or mouth; chronic diseases; medications, dose, and frequency; allergies)

Past Health History (injuries or surgeries of head, eyes, ears, nose, or mouth)

Family History (cancer of mouth or throat, conditions impacting hearing, vision, or thyroid)

Personal and Psychosocial History (last examinations [dental, vision, hearing]; use of assistive devices such as hearing aids, glasses, dentures; use of nicotine and alcohol; health promotion activities: use of protective headgear and eyewear, brushing and flossing practices)

HEALTH PROMOTION AND PROTECTION

1.   Identify risk factors for this patient.

2.   Recommend health promotion activities for this patient.

EXAMINATION

Examination Techniques	Findings (document findings below)
Routine Techniques	
▶ PERFORM hand hygiene.	
Head ▶ INSPECT the head for size, shape, and position.	*Head*
▶ INSPECT skin and scalp for characteristics.	
▶ INSPECT facial structures for size, symmetry, movement, skin characteristics, and facial expressions.	
Techniques for Special Circumstances	
∗ PALPATE the skull for contour, symmetry, tenderness, and intactness.	
∗ PALPATE the bony structures of the face and jaw, noting jaw movement and tenderness.	
∗ PALPATE the temporal arteries for pulsation, texture, and tenderness.	

Examination Techniques	Findings (document findings below)
Routine Techniques	
Eyes	*Eyes*
► TEST visual acuity (distant vision).	Right eye
	Distant vision
	Near vision
► TEST visual acuity (near vision).	Left eye
	Distant vision
	Near vision
	Both eyes
	Distant vision
	Near vision
External Eye	*External Eye*
► ASSESS visual fields for peripheral vision (Confrontation test).	
► INSPECT eyebrows, eyelashes, and eyelids for symmetry, skin characteristics, and discharge.	
► INSPECT conjunctiva for color, drainage, lesions.	
► INSPECT corneal light reflex for symmetry (Hirschberg's test).	
► INSPECT sclera for color and surface characteristics.	

Examination Techniques	Findings (document findings below)
▶ INSPECT cornea for transparency and surface characteristics.	
▶ INSPECT iris for shape and color.	
▶ INSPECT pupils for size, shape, reaction to light, consensual reaction, and accommodation.	
Techniques for Special Circumstances	
✳ ASSESS eye movement for the six cardinal fields of gaze.	
✳ PERFORM cover–uncover eye test.	
✳ PALPATE the eye, eyelids, and lacrimal puncta for firmness, tenderness, and discharge.	
✳ TEST the corneal reflex.	
✳ INSPECT the anterior chamber for transparency, iris surface, and chamber depth.	

Examination Techniques	Findings (document findings below)

Internal Eye
 ✳   INSPECT intraocular structures (ophthalmoscopic examination)
     •   INSPECT for a red reflex.
 	
     •   INSPECT the optic disc for discrete margin, shape, size, color, and physiologic cup.
 	
     •   INSPECT the retinal vessels for color, arteriolar light reflex, artery-to-vein ratio, and arterio-venous crossing changes.
 	
     •   INSPECT the retinal background for color; presence of microaneurysms, hemorrhages, and exudates.
 	
     •   INSPECT the macula for color and surface characteristics.
	Internal Eye

Routine Techniques	
Ear ▶ ASSESS hearing based on response from conversation. ▶ INSPECT the external ears for alignment, position, size, symmetry, skin color, skin intactness, and presence of deformities. ▶ INSPECT the external auditory meatus for discharge or lesions.	*Ear*

Examination Techniques	Findings (document findings below)
Techniques for Special Circumstances	
✱ PALPATE the external ears and mastoid process areas for characteristics, tenderness, and edema.	

✱ INSPECT the internal ear structures.
    • INSPECT the external ear canal for cerumen, odor, edema, erythema, discharge, and foreign bodies.
 	
    • INSPECT the tympanic membrane for landmarks, color, contour, translucence, and fluctuation.	

✱ TEST the acoustic cranial nerve (VIII) to evaluate auditory function.
    • Whispered voice test
 	
    • Finger-rubbing test
 	
    • Weber test
 	
    • Rinne test
 	
    • Audioscope	

Routine Techniques	
Nose ► INSPECT the external nose for appearance, symmetry, and discharge.	*Nose*

Examination Techniques	Findings (document findings below)
Techniques for Special Circumstances	
✳ PALPATE the nose for tenderness and to assess patency.	
✳ INSPECT the internal nasal cavity for surface characteristics, lesions, erythema, discharge, and foreign bodies.	
✳ PALPATE the frontal and maxillary paranasal sinus areas for tenderness.	
✳ TRANSILLUMINATE the sinus area for dim red glow.	
Routine Techniques	
Mouth ▸ INSPECT the lips for color, symmetry, moisture, and texture. ▸ INSPECT the teeth and gums for condition, color, surface characteristics, stability, and alignment. ▸ INSPECT the tongue for movement, symmetry, color, and surface characteristics. ▸ INSPECT the buccal mucosa and anterior and posterior pillars for color, surface characteristics, and odor. ▸ INSPECT the palate, uvula, posterior pharynx, and tonsils for texture, color, surface characteristics, and movement.	*Mouth*

Examination Techniques	Findings (document findings below)
Techniques for Special Circumstances	
✻ PALPATE the teeth, inner lips, and gums for condition and tenderness. ✻ PALPATE the tongue for texture.	
Routine Techniques	
Neck ▶ INSPECT the neck for position in relation to the head and trachea. ▶ INSPECT the neck for skin characteristics and presence of lumps and masses.	*Neck*
Techniques for Special Circumstances	
✻ ESTIMATE range of motion of the neck. ✻ PALPATE the neck for anatomic structures and trachea. *Thyroid* ✻ PALPATE the thyroid gland for size, consistency, tenderness, and presence of nodules.	*Thyroid*
Lymph Nodes ✻ PALPATE lymph nodes for size, consistency, mobility, and tenderness.	*Lymph Nodes*

▶   Routine techniques
✻   Special circumstances

CLINICAL REASONING

1. Organize or cluster your findings data for this patient by body system or concepts.

2. Analyze data collected. (Which data deviate from expected findings? Which additional data are needed?)

3. Determine nursing diagnoses for this patient.

CHAPTER 11 Lungs and Respiratory System

With your lab partner assuming the role of a patient, conduct a focused history and examination. Your "student patient" may role-play a person with a particular respiratory symptom.

HISTORY

BIOGRAPHIC DATA

Date	Name			Gender M F
Date of birth	Age	Race	Marital status S M D W	Occupation

PRESENTING PROBLEM (Check all that apply):

Cough ❑   Shortness of breath ❑   Chest pain with breathing ❑

Other ❑ _____

HISTORY OF PRESENT ILLNESS

Symptom Analysis of Presenting Problem (Onset, Location, Duration, Characteristics, Aggravating and Alleviating factors, Related symptoms, Treatment, Severity)

Present Health Status (chronic diseases; allergies; difficulty breathing; medications, dose, and frequency, or use of oxygen or breathing equipment at home)

Past Health History (problems with lungs or breathing, diagnosed with respiratory disease, injury or surgery to the chest)

Family History (any lung diseases)

Personal and Psychosocial History (tobacco use, home and occupational environments, travel, health promotion practices: handwashing, wearing mask for occupational and environmental respiratory irritants and hazards, annual influenza vaccine, smoking cessation)

HEALTH PROMOTION AND PROTECTION

1. Identify risk factors for this patient.

2. Recommend health promotion activities for this patient.

EXAMINATION

Examination Technique	Findings (document findings below)
Routine Techniques	
► PERFORM hand hygiene.	
► INSPECT the patient for appearance, posture, and breathing effort.	
► COUNT respirations for rate; OBSERVE breathing pattern and chest expansion.	
► INSPECT the patient's nails for color and angle; INSPECT skin and lips for color.	

Examination Technique	Findings (document findings below)
▶ INSPECT the posterior thorax for shape, symmetry, and muscle development.	
▶ AUSCULTATE the posterior and lateral thoraxes for breath sounds.	
▶ INSPECT the anterior thorax for shape, symmetry, muscle development, and costal angle.	
▶ INSPECT anterior thorax for anteroposterior to lateral diameter.	
▶ AUSCULTATE the anterior thorax for breath sounds.	
Techniques for Special Circumstances	
✳ PALPATE posterior and anterior thoracic muscles for tenderness and symmetry.	
✳ PALPATE the posterior and anterior chest walls for thoracic expansion.	
✳ PALPATE the posterior and anterior thoracic walls for vocal (tactile) fremitus.	
✳ PALPATE trachea for position.	

▶ Routine techniques
✳ Techniques for special circumstances

CLINICAL REASONING

1. Organize or cluster your findings for this patient by body system or concepts.

2. Analyze data collected. (Which data deviate from expected findings? Which additional data are needed?)

3. Determine nursing diagnoses for this patient.

CHAPTER 12 Heart and Peripheral Vascular System

With your lab partner assuming the role of a patient, conduct a focused history and examination. Your "student patient" may role-play a person with a particular cardiovascular symptom.

HISTORY

BIOGRAPHIC DATA

Date	Name				Gender M F
Date of birth	Age	Race		Marital status S M D W	Occupation

PRESENTING PROBLEM (Check all that apply):

Chest pain ❑   Shortness of breath ❑   Cough ❑   Urinating during the night ❑

Fatigue ❑   Fainting ❑   Swelling of the extremities ❑   Leg cramps/pain ❑

Other ❑ _____

HISTORY OF PRESENT ILLNESS

Symptom Analysis of Presenting Problem (Onset, Location, Duration, Characteristics, Aggravating and Alleviating factors, Related symptoms, Treatment, Severity)

Present Health Status (chronic diseases; medications, dose, and frequency)

Past Health History (congenital heart disease, high cholesterol or triglycerides, surgeries, electrocardiogram [EKG])

Family History (diabetes, heart disease, hyperlipidemia, or hypertension)

Personal and Psychosocial History (exercise, personality type, relaxation, diet/nutrition, alcohol use, illicit drug use, caffeine intake, smoking, health promotion practices)

HEALTH PROMOTION AND PROTECTION

1.   Identify risk factors for this patient.

2.   Recommend health promotion activities for this patient.

EXAMINATION

Examination Technique	Findings (document findings below)
Routine Techniques	
▸ PERFORM hand hygiene. ▸ INSPECT the patient for general appearance, skin color, and breathing effort.	

Examination Technique	Findings (document findings below)
Peripheral Vascular System ▶ PALPATE temporal and carotid pulses for amplitude. ▶ INSPECT the jugular vein for pulsations. ▶ MEASURE blood pressure. ▶ INSPECT and PALPATE the upper extremities for symmetry and skin turgor. ▶ INSPECT and PALPATE the upper extremities for skin integrity, color, and temperature; capillary refill; and color and angle of nail beds. ▶ PALPATE brachial and radial pulses for rate, rhythm, amplitude, and contour. ▶ INSPECT and PALPATE the lower extremities for symmetry and skin turgor. ▶ INSPECT and PALPATE the lower extremities for skin integrity, color and temperature, capillary refill, hair distribution, color and angle of nail beds, superficial veins, and gross sensation. ▶ PALPATE for femoral, popliteal, posterior tibial, and dorsalis pedis pulses for amplitude.	*Peripheral Vascular System*

Examination Technique	Findings (document findings below)
Heart ▶ INSPECT the anterior chest wall for contour, pulsations, lifts, heaves, and retractions. ▶ PALPATE the apical pulse for location. ▶ AUSCULTATE S_1 and S_2 heart sounds for rate, rhythm, pitch, and splitting. • ASSESS heart rate. • ASSESS rhythm. • ASSESS pitch. • ASSESS splitting. ▶ CALCULATE pulse deficit. ▶ INTERPRET the electrocardiogram.	*Heart*

Examination Technique	Findings (document findings below)
Techniques for Special Circumstances	
Peripheral Vascular System ∗ AUSCULTATE the carotid artery for bruits. ∗ PALPATE epitrochlear lymph nodes for size, consistency, mobility, borders, tenderness, and warmth. ∗ PALPATE inguinal lymph nodes for size, consistency, mobility, borders, tenderness, and warmth. ∗ MEASURE leg circumferences to assess symmetry. ∗ CALCULATE the ankle brachial index (ABI) to estimate arterial occlusion.	*Peripheral Vascular System*

▶ Routine techniques
∗ Special circumstances

CLINICAL REASONING

1. Organize or cluster your findings for this patient by body system or concepts.

2. Analyze data collected. (Which data deviate from expected findings? Which additional data are needed?)

3. Determine nursing diagnoses for this patient.

CHAPTER **13** Abdomen and
Gastrointestinal System

With your lab partner assuming the role of a patient, conduct a focused history and examination. Your "student patient" may role-play a person with a particular abdominal symptom.

HISTORY

BIOGRAPHIC DATA

Date	Name				Gender M F
Date of birth	Age	Race		Marital status S M D W	Occupation

PRESENTING PROBLEM (Check all that apply):

Abdominal pain ❑   Nausea and vomiting ❑   Indigestion ❑   Abdominal distention ❑

Change in bowel habits ❑   Jaundice ❑   Problems with urination ❑

Other ❑ _____

HISTORY OF PRESENT ILLNESS

Symptom Analysis of Presenting Problem (Onset, Location, Duration, Characteristics, Aggravating and Alleviating factors, Related symptoms, Treatment, Severity)

Present Health Status (chronic diseases; medications, dose, and frequency; frequency of bowel movements)

Past Health History (problems with abdomen or digestive system, surgeries of abdomen or urinary tract, problems with the urinary tract or urination)

Family History (history of diseases of the gastrointestinal or urinary systems)

Personal and Psychosocial History (diet/nutrition, alcohol and tobacco use, and health promotion practices: dietary analysis compared to My Plate, use of fiber supplements, and colon cancer screening)

HEALTH PROMOTION AND PROTECTION

1. Identify risk factors for this patient.

2. Recommend health promotion activities for this patient.

EXAMINATION

Examination Technique	Findings (document findings below)
Routine Techniques	
▶ PERFORM hand hygiene.	
▶ OBSERVE the patient's behavior and position.	
▶ INSPECT the abdomen for skin color, surface characteristics, venous patterns, contour, symmetry, and surface movements.	
▶ AUSCULTATE the abdomen for bowel sounds.	

Examination Technique	Findings (document findings below)
▶ AUSCULTATE the abdomen for arterial and venous vascular sounds.	
▶ PALPATE the abdomen lightly for tenderness and muscle tone.	
▶ PALPATE the abdomen deeply for pain, masses, and aortic pulsations.	
Techniques for Special Circumstances	
✳ PERCUSS the abdomen for tones.	
✳ PERCUSS the liver to determine span and descent.	
✳ PERCUSS the spleen for size.	
✳ PALPATE the liver for lower border and pain.	
✳ PALPATE the gallbladder for pain.	
✳ PALPATE the spleen for border and tenderness.	
✳ PALPATE the kidneys for presence, contour, and tenderness.	
✳ PERCUSS the kidneys for costovertebral angle (CVA) tenderness.	

▶   Routine techniques
✳   Special circumstances

CLINICAL REASONING

1. Organize or cluster your findings for this patient by body system or concepts.

2. Analyze the data collected. (Which data deviate from expected findings? Which additional data are needed?)

3. Determine nursing diagnoses for this patient.

CHAPTER 14 Musculoskeletal System

With your lab partner assuming the role of a patient, conduct a focused history and examination. Your "student patient" may role-play a person with a particular musculoskeletal symptom.

HISTORY

BIOGRAPHIC DATA

Date	Name		Gender M F
Date of birth	Age	Race	Marital status S M D W	Occupation

PRESENTING PROBLEM (Check all that apply):

Pain ❏   Problems with movement ❏

Problems with daily activities ❏

    Bathing ❏   Eating ❏   Toileting ❏   Moving around ❏

    Dressing ❏   Communicating ❏   Grooming ❏

Other ❏ _____

HISTORY OF PRESENT ILLNESS

Symptom Analysis of Presenting Problem (Onset, Location, Duration, Characteristics, Aggravating and Alleviating factors, Related symptoms, Treatment, Severity)

Present Health Status (chronic diseases; medications, dose, and frequency; any changes in your ability to move around)

Past Health History (accidents/injuries or surgeries)

Family History (curvature of the spine or back problems; rheumatoid arthritis, osteoarthritis, or gout)

Personal and Psychosocial History (alcohol use, protection from muscle strain or injury, health promotion practices: type, frequency, and duration of exercise; calcium intake; and osteoporosis screening)

HEALTH PROMOTION AND PROTECTION

1. Identify risk factors for this patient.

2. Recommend health promotion activities for this patient.

EXAMINATION

Examination Technique	Findings (document findings below)
Routine Techniques	
► PERFORM hand hygiene.	
► INSPECT skeleton and extremities for alignment and symmetry.	
► INSPECT muscles for symmetry and size.	

Examination Technique	Findings (document findings below)
▶ PALPATE bones for pain; joints for pain, temperature, and edema; and muscles for pain, temperature, edema, and tone.	
▶ OBSERVE range of motion for major joints and adjacent muscles, for pain on movement, joint stability, and deformity.	
▶ TEST muscle strength and compare sides.	
As needed, examine any or all of the following specific body regions	
▶ OBSERVE gait for conformity, symmetry, and rhythm.	
Head and Neck ▶ INSPECT musculature of the face and neck for symmetry.	*Head and Neck*
▶ PALPATE each temporomandibular joint for movement, pain, and sounds.	
▶ OBSERVE jaw for range of motion. • Open and close	
• Side to side	
• Protrude and retract	
▶ PALPATE the neck for tone.	

Examination Technique	Findings (document findings below)
► OBSERVE the neck for range of motion. • Flexion and hyperextension • Lateral bending • Rotation ► TEST neck muscles for strength.	
Upper Body (neck, spine, shoulders, extremities) ► INSPECT the shoulders and cervical, thoracic, and lumbar spine for alignment and symmetry. ► OBSERVE range of motion of the thoracic and lumbar spine. • Flexion and hyperextension • Lateral bending • Rotation ► PALPATE the posterior neck, spinal processes, and paravertebral muscles for alignment and pain. ► PERCUSS the spinal processes for pain. ► INSPECT the shoulders and shoulder girdle for equality of height, symmetry, and contour.	***Upper Body***

Examination Technique	Findings (document findings below)
▶ PALPATE the shoulders for firmness, fullness, symmetry, and pain.	
▶ TEST the trapezius muscles for strength.	
▶ OBSERVE the shoulders for range of motion and symmetry. NOTICE any crepitation or report of pain. • Extension and hyperextension • Abduction and adduction • External rotation • Internal rotation	
▶ TEST the arms for muscle strength.	
▶ PALPATE the elbows for pain, edema, temperature, and nodules.	
▶ OBSERVE the elbows for range of motion. • Flexion and extension • Supination and pronation	
▶ INSPECT the joints of the wrists and hands for symmetry, alignment, and number of digits.	
▶ PALPATE each joint of the hand and wrist for surface characteristics and pain.	
▶ TEST for muscle strength of fingers and grip.	

Examination Technique	Findings (document findings below)

► OBSERVE for range of motion of wrists and fingers.
  • Wrist flexion and hyperextension
 	
  • Metacarpophalangeal flexion and hyperextension
 	
  • Wrist radial and ulnar deviation
 	
  • Finger abduction
 	
  • Finger flexion, fist formation
 	
  • Finger extension, thumb to each fingertip, to base of little finger	

Lower Body (Hips, knees, extremities)
► INSPECT the hips for symmetry.
 	
► PALPATE the hips for stability and pain.
 	
► OBSERVE the hips for range of motion.
  • Hip flexion, knee flexion
 	
  • Hip flexion leg extension
 	
  • External and internal hip rotation
 	
  • Hip abduction and adduction
 	
  • Hip hyperextension, leg extended
	Lower Body

Examination Technique	Findings (document findings below)
► TEST the hips for muscle strength.	
► TEST the leg muscles for strength.	
► INSPECT the knees for symmetry and alignment.	
► PALPATE the knees for contour.	
► OBSERVE the knees for range of motion. 　• Flexion and hyperextension	
► INSPECT the ankles and feet for contour, number of toes, alignment, and deformity.	
► PALPATE the ankles and feet for contour.	
► OBSERVE the ankles and feet for range of motion. 　• Dorsiflexion and plantar flexion 　• Inversion and eversion 　• Abduction and adduction 　• Flex and extend the toes	
► TEST the ankle and foot muscles for strength.	
Techniques for Special Circumstances	
✳ ASSESS for nerve root compression.	

► Routine techniques
✳ Special circumstances

CLINICAL REASONING

1. Organize or cluster your findings for this patient by body system or concepts.

2. Analyze data collected. (Which data deviate from expected findings? Which additional data are needed?)

3. Determine nursing diagnoses for this patient.

CHAPTER **15** Neurologic System

With your lab partner assuming the role of a patient, conduct a focused history and examination. Your "student patient" may role-play a person with a particular neurologic symptom.

HISTORY

BIOGRAPHIC DATA

Date	Name				Gender M F
Date of birth	Age	Race		Marital status S M D W	Occupation

PRESENTING PROBLEM (Check all that apply):

Headaches ❏   Seizures ❏   Loss of consciousness ❏   Changes in movement ❏

Changes in sensation ❏   Difficulty swallowing ❏   Difficulty communicating ❏

Other ❏ _____

HISTORY OF PRESENT ILLNESS

Symptom Analysis of Presenting Problem (Onset, Location, Duration, Characteristics, Aggravating and Alleviating factors, Related symptoms, Treatment, Severity)

Present Health Status (any changes in ability to move around; chronic conditions that affect mobility; and medications, dose, and frequency)

Past Health History (injury to head or spinal cord; surgery of brain, spinal cord, or nerves; or history of stroke or seizures)

Family History (history of stroke, seizure, or brain tumor)

Personal and Psychosocial History (functional ability, alcohol and illicit drug use, and health promotion activities: use of helmet when biking and use of seat beats)

HEALTH PROMOTION AND PROTECTION

1. Identify risk factors for this patient.

2. Recommend health promotion activities for this patient.

EXAMINATION

Examination Technique	Findings (document findings below)
Routine Techniques	
► PERFORM hand hygiene.	
► ASSESS mental status and level of consciousness.	
► EVALUATE speech for articulation and voice quality and conversation for comprehension of verbal communication.	

Examination Technique	Findings (document findings below)

▶ NOTICE cranial nerve functions.
  • CN I (olfactory)—smell
 	
  • CN II (optic nerve)—sight
 	
  • CN III (oculomotor), IV (trochlear), VI (abducens)—eye movement
 	
  • CN V (trigeminal)—eye blink
 	
  • CN VII (facial)—symmetric face
 	
  • CN VIII (acoustic)—hearing
 	
  • CN IX (glossopharyngeal), CN X (vagus)—swallowing and ability to handle saliva
 	
  • CN X (vagus)—guttural speech sounds
 	
  • CN XI (spinal accessory)—shrug shoulders or turn head
 	
▶ OBSERVE gait for balance and symmetry.
 	
▶ EVALUATE extremities for muscle strength and tone.	

Examination Technique	Findings (document findings below)
Techniques for Special Circumstances	

✳ ASSESS individual cranial nerves.
   • TEST nose for smell.
 	
   • TEST eyes for visual acuity.
 	
   • TEST eyes for peripheral vision.
 	
   • OBSERVE eyes for extraocular muscle movement.
 	
   • OBSERVE eyes for pupillary size, shape, equality, constriction, and accommodation.
 	
   • EVALUATE face for movement and sensation.
 	
   • TEST ears for hearing.
 	
   • TEST tongue for taste.
 	
   • INSPECT oropharynx for gag reflex and movement of soft palate.
 	
   • TEST tongue for movement, symmetry, strength, and absence of tumors.
 	
   • TEST shoulders and neck muscles for strength, movement, and symmetry.	

Examination Technique	Findings (document findings below)

✳ TEST cerebellar function for balance and coordination. (Use at least two techniques.)
  • TEST for balance.
    – Romberg test
 	
    – With eyes closed, stand on one foot, then the other
 	
    – Heel-to-toe walking
 	
    – Hop on one foot, then the other
 	
    – Deep knee bends
 	
    – Walk on toes, then on heels
 	
  • EVALUATE upper extremity coordination.
    – Alternately tap hands to thighs
 	
    – With eyes closed and outstretched arms, touch finger to own nose
 	
    – Touch each finger to thumb in rapid sequence
 	
    – Rapidly move finger between nose and nurse's finger
 	
  • EVALUATE lower extremity coordination.
    – Lying supine, slide heel down opposite shin	

Examination Technique	Findings (document findings below)

✳ ASSESS sensory function.
  • ASSESS sensation to light touch.
 	
  • ASSESS sharp and dull sensation.
 	
  • ASSESS vibratory sense using tuning fork.
 	
  • ASSESS kinesthetic sensation or test of proprioception.
 	
  • TEST stereognosis.
 	
  • TEST two-point discrimination.
 	
  • TEST for extinction.
 	
  • EVALUATE graphesthesia.
 	
  • TEST point location.
 	
  • ASSESS peripheral sensation using a monofilament.	

Examination Technique	Findings (document findings below)

✳ EVALUATE extremities for deep tendon reflexes.
    • Triceps reflex
 	
    • Biceps reflex
 	
    • Brachioradial reflex
 	
    • Patellar reflex
 	
    • Achilles tendon
 	
 ✳ EVALUATE plantar reflex.
 	
 ✳ EVALUATE ankle clonus.	

▶   Routine techniques
✳   Special circumstances

CLINICAL REASONING

1. Organize or cluster your findings for this patient by body system or concepts.

2. Analyze data collected. (Which data deviate from expected findings? Which additional data are needed?)

3. Determine nursing diagnoses for this patient.

Student Name_____   Date_____

CHAPTER 16 Breasts and Axillae

With your lab partner assuming the role of a patient, conduct a focused history and examination. Your "student patient" may role-play a person with a particular symptom associated with the breasts. Your lab may have a breast model that can be used to learn the examination.

HISTORY

BIOGRAPHIC DATA

Date	Name			Gender M F
Date of birth	Age	Race	Marital status S M D W	Occupation

PRESENTING PROBLEM (Check all that apply):

Breast pain/tenderness ❑   Breast lump ❑   Nipple discharge ❑   Axillary lumps/tenderness ❑

Breast swelling or enlargement (men) ❑   Other ❑

HISTORY OF PRESENT ILLNESS

Symptom Analysis of Presenting Problem (Onset, Location, Duration, Characteristics, Aggravating and Alleviating factors, Related symptoms, Treatment, Severity)

Present Health Status (medications, dose, and frequency; intake of chocolate and caffeine)

Past Health History (problem with breasts such as fibrocystic changes, fibroadenoma, breast cancer; history of ovarian cancer, endometrial cancer, or colon cancer; any surgery on breasts; date of menarche and menopause)

Family History (history of breast cancer in the family)

Personal and Psychosocial History (breast examination, mammogram, alcohol use, health promotion practices)

HEALTH PROMOTION AND PROTECTION

1. Identify risk factors for this patient.

2. Recommend health promotion activities for this patient.

EXAMINATION

Examination Technique	Findings (document findings below)
Female Breast	**Female Breast**
Routine Techniques	
▶ PERFORM hand hygiene.	
▶ INSPECT breasts for size, shape, and symmetry.	
▶ INSPECT the skin of the breasts for color, surface characteristics, and venous patterns.	
▶ INSPECT the areolae for color, shape, and surface characteristics.	
▶ INSPECT the nipples for position, symmetry, surface characteristics, lesions, bleeding, and discharge.	

Examination Technique	Findings (document findings below)
Techniques for Special Circumstances	
✳ INSPECT the breasts in various positions for bilateral pull, symmetry, and contour.	
✳ INSPECT and PALPATE the axillae for enlarged lymph nodes, rash, lesions, or masses.	
✳ PALPATE the breasts for tissue characteristics.	
✳ PALPATE the nipples for surface characteristics and discharge.	
Male Breast	**Male Breast**
Routine Techniques	
▶ PERFORM hand hygiene.	
▶ INSPECT the breasts, nipples, and areolae for symmetry, color, size, shape, rash, and lesions.	
Techniques for Special Circumstances	
✳ PALPATE the breasts and nipples for surface characteristics, tenderness, size, and masses.	
✳ PALPATE the axillae for lymph nodes.	

▶ Routine techniques
✳ Special circumstances

CLINICAL REASONING

1. Organize or cluster your findings for this patient by body system or concepts.

2. Analyze data collected. (Which data deviate from expected findings? Which additional data are needed?)

3. Determine nursing diagnoses for this patient.

CHAPTER **17** Reproductive System and the Perineum

With your lab partner assuming the role of a patient, conduct a focused history and examination. Your "student patient" may role-play a person with a particular symptom. Your lab may have a model that can be used to learn the examination.

HISTORY

BIOGRAPHIC DATA

Date	Name		Gender M F
Date of birth	Age	Race	Marital status S M D W	Occupation

PRESENTING PROBLEM (Check all that apply):

Female

Pain ❑   Genital lesions ❑   Vaginal discharge ❑

Problems with menstruation ❑   Menopausal symptoms ❑   Rectal bleeding ❑

Other ❑

Male

Pain ❑   Genital lesions ❑   Penile discharge ❑

Difficulty with erection ❑   Problems with urination ❑   Rectal bleeding ❑

Other ❑

HISTORY OF PRESENT ILLNESS

Symptom Analysis of Presenting Problem (Onset, Location, Duration, Characteristics, Aggravating and Alleviating factors, Related symptoms, Treatment, Severity)

Present Health Status (chronic conditions; medications, dose, and frequency)

Past Health History (reproductive problems, surgeries, history of cancer, immunizations [hepatitis A, hepatitis B, human papillomavirus])

Family History (females: cancer of cervix, ovary, uterus, breast, or colon; males: cancer of prostate or testicles)

Personal and Psychosocial History (self-examination of genitalia, exam by health professional, health promotion practices: methods to prevent unwanted pregnancies and protection from sexually transmitted diseases)

Sexual history (number of partners, protection from STDs, and birth control)

Women:

Obstetric history

Menstruation (date of last menstrual period, how often are menstrual periods, any changes in periods, age at first menstrual period)

Pregnancy (number of pregnancies; number of abortions, miscarriages, or fetuses that died before birth; any difficulty becoming pregnant)

HEALTH PROMOTION AND PROTECTION

1. Identify risk factors for this patient.

2. Recommend health promotion activities for this patient.

EXAMINATION

Examination Technique	Findings (document findings below)
Routine Techniques	
Female ▶ PERFORM hand hygiene and don examination gloves. ▶ INSPECT the pubic hair and skin over the mons pubis and inguinal area for distribution and surface characteristics. ▶ INSPECT and PALPATE the labia majora, labia minora, and clitoris for pigmentation and surface characteristics. ▶ INSPECT the urethral meatus, vaginal introitus, and perineum for positioning and surface characteristics. ▶ INSPECT and PALPATE the sacrococcygeal areas for surface characteristics and tenderness. ▶ INSPECT the perianal area and anus for color and surface characteristics.	*Female*

Examination Technique	Findings (document findings below)
Techniques for Special Circumstances	
* PALPATE the Skene and Bartholin glands for surface characteristics, discharge, and pain or discomfort.	
* PALPATE the vaginal wall for tone.	
* PALPATE the rectal wall for surface characteristics.	
* PALPATE the anal sphincter for muscle tone.	
* EXAMINE stool for characteristics and presence of occult blood.	

▶ Routine techniques
* Special circumstances

Examination Technique	Findings (document findings below)
Routine Techniques	
Male	*Male*
▶ PERFORM hand hygiene and don examination gloves.	
▶ INSPECT the pubic hair for distribution and skin for general characteristics.	
▶ INSPECT and PALPATE the penis for surface characteristics, color, tenderness, and discharge.	
▶ INSPECT the scrotum for color, texture, surface characteristics, and position.	

Examination Technique	Findings (document findings below)
▶ INSPECT the inguinal region and the femoral area for bulges.	
▶ INSPECT and PALPATE the sacrococcygeal areas for surface characteristics and tenderness.	
▶ INSPECT the perianal area and anus for pigmentation and surface characteristics.	
Techniques for Special Circumstances	
✳ PALPATE scrotum for surface characteristics and tenderness.	
✳ PALPATE the testes, epididymides, and vasa deferentia for location, consistency, tenderness, and nodules.	
✳ PALPATE the anus for sphincter tone.	
✳ PALPATE the anal canal and rectum for surface characteristics.	
✳ EXAMINE stool for characteristics and presence of occult blood.	

▶   Routine techniques
✳   Special circumstances

CLINICAL REASONING

1. Organize or cluster your findings for this patient by body system or concepts.

2. Analyze data collected. (Which data deviate from expected findings? Which additional data are needed?)

3. Determine nursing diagnoses for this patient.

CHAPTER 18 Developmental Assessment Throughout the Life Span

No laboratory activities are required for the content in this chapter.

CHAPTER 19   Assessment of the Infant, Child, and Adolescent

With your lab partner assuming the role of the patient's parent or with an actual child or infant patient, conduct a focused history and examination. Your "student parent" may role-play the parent of a child with a particular symptom. Your lab may have a model that can be used to learn the examination.

HISTORY

BIOGRAPHIC DATA

Date	Name				Gender M F
Date of birth	Age	Race		Marital status S M D W	Occupation

REASON FOR SEEKING HEALTH CARE (Presenting Problem)

HISTORY OF PRESENT ILLNESS

Symptom Analysis of Presenting Problem (Onset, Location, Duration, Characteristics, Aggravating and Alleviating factors, Related symptoms, Treatment, Severity)

Present Health Status

Current Health Conditions

Current medications: Prescription/Over-the-Counter/Herbal (Document if no medications are taken)

Name of Drug	Dosage/Frequency	Last Dose Taken	Reason for Taking

Allergies: Medication/Food/Other (latex, contrast, iodine) (Document if there are no allergies)

Allergic To	Type of Reaction

Current Medical Treatments:

Treatment Modality	Reason for Treatment

PAST HEALTH HISTORY

Mother's health status and pregnancy history (for newborns, infants, toddlers, and older children with chronic health problems only) (See Box 19-2), childhood illnesses, immunizations, and last examinations:

Pregnancy

History	Considerations	Findings
Prenatal care	Care received, complications, bleeding problems, hypertension, edema, proteinuria, weight gain, infections, gestational diabetes, preterm labor	
Substance use during pregnancy	Alcohol, tobacco, medications, street drugs	
Mother's emotional state during pregnancy	Anxiety, depression, acceptance of pregnancy, mental health issues	
Labor and delivery process	Place of birth (hospital, home, birth center)	
Mother's labor	Spontaneous, induced, duration, medications, complications	
Infant delivery	Vaginal, cesarean section, use of anesthesia, special equipment and procedures	

Newborn Course

History	Considerations	Findings
Birth history	Gestational age and growth pattern	
Apgar	Apgar score and type of resuscitation if required	
Neonatal complications	Respiratory, infections, feeding, hyperbilirubinemia, congenital abnormalities	

Childhood Illnesses (Check all that apply):

Measles ❑   Mumps ❑   Rubella ❑   Chickenpox ❑

Pertussis ❑   Influenza ❑   Otitis media ❑   Streptococcal throat infections ❑

Other ❑

	Description	Date / Year	Residual Problems
Previous medical conditions			
Previous hospitalizations			
Injuries			
Surgeries			

Immunizations

	Recommended Administration Schedule (not absolute)	Date Given		Reactions
Hepatitis B virus (HBV)	3 doses between birth and 18 months	Dose 1		
		Dose 2		
		Dose 3		
Rotavirus (RV)	3 doses between 2 and 6 months	Dose 1		
		Dose 2		
		Dose 3		
Diphtheria and tetanus toxoid and acellular pertussis (DTaP)	4 doses between 4 weeks and 18 months Booster at 4 to 6 years	Dose 1		
		Dose 2		
		Dose 3		
		Dose 4		
		Booster		
Haemophilus influenza type b conjugate (Hib)	Up to 4 doses from 2 months to 18 months (varies)	Dose 1		
		Dose 2		
		Dose 3		
		Dose 4		
Inactivated poliovirus (IPV)	3 doses between 2 and 18 months Booster at 4 to 6 years	Dose 1		
		Dose 2		
		Dose 3		
		Booster		
Pneumococcal conjugate vaccine (PCV13)	3 doses from 2 months to 18 months	Dose 1		
		Dose 2		
		Dose 3		
Measles, mumps, rubella (MMR)	2 doses between 12 and 15 months and 4 and 6 years	Dose 1		
		Dose 2		
Varicella	2 doses between 12 to 15 months and 4 to 6 years	Dose 1		
		Dose 2		
Hepatitis A virus (HBA)	1 dose at 12 to 23 months	Dose 1		
Tetanus, diphtheria, pertussis (Tdap)	1 dose between ages 11 and 12	Dose 1		
Human papilloma virus (HPV)	3 doses between 11 and 12 years	Dose 1		
		Dose 2		
		Dose 3		
Meningococcal conjugate vaccine (MCV)	1 dose between 11 to 12 years	Dose 1		
Influenza	Annually after age 6 months			

Date of Last Examination

Physical Examination: _____   Vision Examination: _____

Hearing Examination: _____   Dental Examination: _____

FAMILY HISTORY (Indicate age and current health. If deceased, indicate age and cause of death.)

Person	Age	Current Health	Person	Age	Current Health
Mother			Father		
Maternal Grandfather			Paternal Grandfather		
Maternal Grandmother			Paternal Grandmother		
Aunt / Uncle			Aunt / Uncle		
Aunt / Uncle			Aunt / Uncle		
Sister			Brother		
Sister			Brother		

PERSONAL AND PSYCHOSOCIAL HISTORY

Personal Status (personality, temperament, habits, rituals)

Nutrition and Diet (typical diet and food preferences, allergies, tolerances, supplements, habits related to food or eating [e.g., bottles in bed])

Sleep (where child sleeps, hours per night, naps, parent challenges)

Sexuality (older child history of development and concerns)

Development (review milestones and record concerns)

Health Promotion Activities (exercise, television time, computer time, alcohol, drugs, smoking, injury prevention such as bicycle helmets, car seats)

Social and Family Relationships (family composition, family life, family socioeconomic status, home environment, and friends)

Mental Health (coping, ability to settle self, school performance, mood)

REVIEW OF SYSTEMS (Check all symptoms that apply, add comment below)

General Symptoms			
Fevers ❑	Night sweats ❑	Pain ❑	Fatigue ❑
Change in energy level ❑	Activity intolerance ❑	Problems sleeping ❑	Unexplained changes in weight ❑
Comments:			

Integumentary System

Change in skin color/ texture ❑	Easy bruising ❑	Piercings and tattoos ❑	Skin lesions ❑
Skin dryness or scaling ❑	Skin itching/irritation ❑	Sores that do not heal ❑	Nail biting ❑
Hair (infestations) ❑	Seborrhea ❑	Recent hair loss ❑	Change in nails ❑
Comments:			

Head

Head size and shape ❑	Headaches ❑	Recent trauma ❑	
Comments:			

Eyes

Not fixing on objects (infants) ❑	Difficulty reading ❑	Abnormal eye movement ❑	Eye pain ❑
Drainage or crusting ❑	Sitting too close to computer screen ❑	Redness ❑	Eye itching ❑
Wear corrective lenses? ❑	If yes:	How long?	Last date evaluated?
Comments:			

Ears

Ear pain ❑	Drainage ❑	Concerns about hearing ❑	Loud speech ❑
Comments:			

Nose			
Nasal congestion ❑	Frequent nosebleeds ❑	Sneezing ❑	Snoring ❑
Comments:			

Mouth/Throat			
Throat pain ❑	Mouth pain or lesions ❑	Coating on tongue ❑	Teeth (tooth loss, caries, pain) ❑
Change in voice ❑	Trouble swallowing ❑		
Comments:			

Neck			
Lymph node enlargement ❑	Swelling or mass in neck ❑	Stiff neck ❑	Unusual position of head/neck ❑
Comments:			

Breasts			
Breast engorgement (newborns) ❑	Pain ❑	Breast changes (developmental) ❑	
Comments:			

Respiratory System			
Cough ❑	Shortness of breath ❑	Wheezing ❑	Snoring ❑
Increased respiratory rate or effort ❑			
Comments:			

Cardiovascular System

Cyanosis or pallor ❑	Edema ❑	Known murmur ❑	Syncope ❑
Comments:			

Gastrointestinal System

Unusual pattern of bowel movements ❑	Constipation ❑	Diarrhea ❑	Abdominal pain ❑
Change in appetite ❑	Nausea/vomiting ❑		
Comments:			

Urinary System

Number of wet diapers ❑	Toilet training ❑	Enuresis ❑	Dysuria, frequency ❑
Comments:			

Reproductive System

Boys

Circumcision ❑	Rash ❑	Pain ❑	Itching ❑
Trauma ❑	Secondary sex characteristics ❑	Testicular masses ❑	

Girls

Menstrual concerns ❑	Rash ❑	Trauma ❑	Secondary sex characteristics ❑
Comments:			

Musculoskeletal System

Muscle pain ❑	Joint pain ❑	Asymmetric movement ❑	Injury history ❑
Spine curvature ❑	Limitations in range of motion ❑	Deformity of legs ❑	
Comments:			

Neurologic System			
Unusual cry ❑	Irritability ❑	Speech problems ❑	Seizures ❑
Fainting/dizziness ❑	Difficulty with coordination and gait ❑		
Comments:			

EXAMINATION

Perform techniques appropriate for the age of the child being examined.

Examination Technique	Findings (document findings below)
▶ PERFORM hand hygiene. *Vital Signs and Baseline Measurement* ▶ MEASURE vital signs. ▶ MEASURE height and weight.	*Vital Signs and Baseline Measurement* Temperature: Heart rate: Blood pressure: Respiratory rate: Height/Length: Weight:
Skin ▶ INSPECT skin for color, birthmarks, lesions, and turgor.	*Skin*

Examination Technique	Findings (document findings below)
Hair and Nails ► INSPECT scalp for texture. ► INSPECT hair for quality, distribution, cleanliness, infestations. ► INSPECT NAILS for shape, consistency, and color.	**Hair and Nails**
Head ► MEASURE head circumference. ► INSPECT the head for skin characteristics, pigmentation, and edema. ► (Infant) PALPATE fontanels for concavity.	**Head**

Examination Technique	Findings (document findings below)
Eyes ► SCREEN for visual acuity. ► INSPECT eyelids for edema, epicanthal folds, and position. ► NOTICE the alignment and slant of the palpebral fissures (see Fig. 10-13 and Fig. 19-18). ► OBSERVE for wide-spaced eyes. ► INSPECT sclera for color. ► INSPECT eye movement in six cardinal fields of gaze. ► OBSERVE for pupillary reaction. ► ASSESS for corneal light reflex. ► VISUALIZE the red reflex.	*Eyes*

Examination Technique	Findings (document findings below)
Ears ► SCREEN for hearing. ► INSPECT the external ears for symmetry and position in relation to outer canthus of the eye. ► INSPECT external ear canal and tympanic membrane for color and characteristics.	*Ears*
Nose and Mouth ► INSPECT nose for size and patency. ► PALPATE sinuses. ► INSPECT mouth for color, moisture, lesions, and intactness. ► ASSESS suck in infants (with gloved hand). ► INSPECT teeth for presence, hygiene, and characteristics. ► INSPECT posterior pharynx and gag reflex.	*Nose and Mouth*

Examination Technique	Findings (document findings below)
Neck ► ASSESS for head lag in infants. ► INSPECT the neck for a midline trachea, abnormal skinfolds, and neck enlargement. ✳ PALPATE for tone, presence of masses, and enlarged lymph nodes. ✳ INSPECT and PALPATE thyroid.	**Neck**
Lungs and Respiratory System ► INSPECT the chest for respiratory effort. ► MEASURE chest circumference. ► INSPECT the anterior and posterior chest for symmetry and ease of respirations. ► INSPECT the anterior-posterior to lateral diameter of the chest. ► AUSCULTATE the anterior, lateral, and posterior chest for lung sounds. ✳ PALPATE thoracic muscles for symmetry, pain, and bulges.	**Lungs and Respiratory System**

Examination Technique	Findings (document findings below)
Heart and Peripheral Vascular System ▶ ASSESS the pulses including rate, rhythm, and characteristics. May be apical in the infant and radial in the older child. ▶ INSPECT and PALPATE the chest for size, shape, and abnormal pulsations. ▶ AUSCULTATE heart for sounds. ▶ AUSCULTATE for venous hum. ▶ ASSESS for capillary refill.	*Heart and Peripheral Vascular System*
Abdomen and Gastrointestinal System ▶ INSPECT for symmetry, color, surface characteristics, and movement. ▶ INSPECT the newborn's umbilicus for color and arteries and a vein. ▶ PALPATE the abdomen for characteristics and softness. ▶ AUSCULTATE the abdomen for bowel sounds.	*Abdomen and Gastrointestinal System*

Examination Technique	Findings (document findings below)
Musculoskeletal System ▶ INSPECT development appropriate for age. (See Tables 18-3, 18-4, and 18-5) ▶ INSPECT gait for balance and coordination. ▶ INSPECT shoulders, scapulas, and iliac crests for symmetry. ▶ INSPECT back and spine for alignment, tufts of hair, and bulges. ▶ ASSESS all muscles for tone. ▶ OBSERVE range of motion. ▶ (Infant) PALPATE and MANIPULATE hips for clicking and integrity.	***Musculoskeletal System***

Examination Technique	Findings (document findings below)
Neurologic System (Palpating fontelles and measuring head circumference performed earlier are part of the neurologic assessment.) ▶ OBSERVE spontaneous motor activity for symmetry. ▶ NOTICE the infant's quality of cry. ▶ OBSERVE infant's response to touch. ▶ INSPECT development appropriate for age. (See Tables 18-3, 18-4, and 18-5) ▶ (Infant) INSPECT infantile reflexes. (See Table 19-4) ✳ ASSESS for neurologic soft signs. (See Table 19-5) ✳ ASSESS cranial nerves appropriate for age. ✳ TEST extremities for superficial tactile sensation. ✳ TEST the reflexes. • Deep tendon reflexes • Babinski reflex • Ankle clonus	*Neurologic System*
Breast ▶ INSPECT the breasts for characteristics.	*Breast*

Examination Technique	Findings (document findings below)
Reproductive System and Perineum ▶ Don examination gloves. ▶ INSPECT the external genitalia. 　• Female: the genitalia, the urethra, the clitoris, the hymen, and the vaginal opening for characteristics. 　• Male: the penis, foreskin, and scrotum for characteristics. ▶ PALPATE the scrotum to determine presence of the testes.	*Reproductive System and Perineum*
Perianal ▶ INSPECT the anus for color and surface characteristics.	*Perianal*

▶　Routine techniques
＊　Special circumstances

CLINICAL REASONING

1. Organize or cluster your findings for this patient by body system or concepts.

2. Analyze data collected. (Which data deviate from expected findings? Which additional data are needed?)

3. Determine nursing diagnoses for this patient.

CHAPTER **20** Assessment of the Pregnant Patient

With your lab partner assuming the role of a patient, conduct a history and examination. Your "student patient" may role-play a person with a particular symptom.

HISTORY

BIOGRAPHIC DATA

Date	Name				Gender M F
Date of birth	Age	Race		Marital status S M D W	Occupation

PRESENTING PROBLEM

HISTORY OF PRESENT ILLNESS

Symptom Analysis of Presenting Problem (Onset, Location, Duration, Characteristics, Aggravating and Alleviating factors, Related symptoms, Treatment, Severity)

Present Health Status (chronic health conditions; medications, dose, and frequency)

Past Health History (surgeries, hospitalizations, accidents, immunizations)

Gynecologic Obstetric History (GTPAL)

Last menstrual period (LMP): _____   Gravidity: _____   Term births: _____

Preterm births: _____   Abortions/miscarriages: _____   Living children: _____

Description of Previous Pregnancies

- Course of pregnancy

- Process of labor

- Delivery

- Condition of infant at birth

- Postpartum course

- Fertility interventions

Family History (multiple births, chromosome abnormalities, genetic disorders, congenital disorders, and chronic illnesses such as diabetes mellitus, renal disease, or cancer)

PERSONAL AND PSYCHOSOCIAL HISTORY

Attitude Toward Pregnancy: (feelings about pregnancy, was pregnancy planned, expectations of pregnancy, pregnancy fears, expectations of parent role, emotional stability)

Diet/Nutrition: (usual dietary practices, food allergies and intolerances, lactose intolerance, ingestion of nonnutritive substances)

Tobacco, Alcohol, and Illicit Drug Use: (amount used and frequency)

Environment: (safety at home and work, seatbelt use, report of domestic violence or abuse, physical abuse, feelings of not being safe)

REVIEW OF SYSTEMS (same as for adult patient plus pregnancy-related review)

Specific Pregnancy-Related Review of Systems:

Fetal Assessment:
Report of fetal movement ❑   Time of day _____   Frequency _____

Integumentary System:
Skin marks, lines, and varicosities ❑   Pruritus ❑

Nose and Mouth:
Nose bleeding or stuffiness ❑   Gum bleeding or swelling ❑

Ears:
Changes in hearing ❑   Sense of fullness in ears ❑

Eyes:
Excessive dryness ❑   Visual changes ❑

Respiratory System:
Shortness of breath ❑

Cardiovascular System:
Palpitations ❑   Edema of extremities ❑   Orthostatic hypotension (dizziness when standing up) ❑

Breasts:
Enlargement, engorgement, tenderness ❑   Nipple discharge ❑

Gastrointestinal System:
Nausea, vomiting (morning sickness) ❑   Loss of appetite ❑   Food aversions ❑
Heartburn (gastric reflux) ❑   Epigastric pain (second and third trimester) ❑
Constipation (second and third trimester) ❑   Hemorrhoids (second and third trimester) ❑

Genitourinary System:
Urinary pain, frequency, and urgency ❑   Vaginal discharge or bleeding ❑

Musculoskeletal System:
Backache ❑   Leg cramps ❑

Neurologic System:
Headaches ❑

HEALTH PROMOTION AND PROTECTION

1. Identify risk factors for this patient.

2. Recommend health promotion activities for this patient.

EXAMINATION

Examination Technique	Findings (document findings below)
▶ PERFORM hand hygiene.	
Vital Signs, Height, and Weight ▶ MEASURE temperature, blood pressure, pulse, and respirations.	***Measurements*** Temperature: Heart rate: Blood pressure: Respiratory rate:
▶ MEASURE height and weight.	Height: Weight:
▶ Determine BMI.	BMI:
Extremities ▶ INSPECT the hands and nails for color, surface characteristics, edema, movement, and sensation. ▶ INSPECT and PALPATE the lower extremities for edema, surface characteristics, redness, and tenderness.	***Extremities***

Examination Technique	Findings (document findings below)
Head, Eyes, Ears, Nose, and Throat ▶ INSPECT the head and face for skin characteristics, pigmentation, and edema. ▶ INSPECT the eyes and TEST vision for acuity. ▶ INSPECT the ears, nose, and mouth as described in Chapter 10. ▶ INSPECT and PALPATE the neck as described in Chapter 10.	***Head, Eyes, Ears, Nose, and Throat***
Anterior and Posterior Chest ▶ INSPECT, PALPATE, and AUSCULTATE the anterior and posterior chest, as described in Chapters 11 and 12.	***Anterior and Posterior Chest***
Breast ▶ INSPECT and PALPATE the breasts for surface and tissue characteristics. ▶ INSPECT and PALPATE the nipples for surface characteristics and nipple shape.	***Breast***
Musculoskeletal ▶ INSPECT and PALPATE the spine, extremities, and joints as described in Chapter 14. ▶ INSPECT posture and gait.	***Musculoskeletal***

Examination Technique	Findings (document findings below)
Neurologic ▶ EXAMINE the patient for neurologic changes.	*Neurologic*
Abdomen ▶ INSPECT for surface characteristics and fetal movement. ▶ MEASURE the fundus for height. ▶ AUSCULTATE for fetal heart sounds. ∗ PALPATE for fetal movement and uterine contraction. ∗ PALPATE fetal position for fetal lie and presentation, position, and attitude.	*Abdomen* Fundal height: _____ cm Fetal heart sounds: _____/min
Genitalia ▶ INSPECT the external genitalia for appearance and discharge. ∗ PALPATE the cervix to determine length (effacement) and dilation.	*Genitalia*
Anus and Rectum ▶ INSPECT and PALPATE the anus and rectum for hemorrhoids.	*Anus and Rectum*

▶   Routine techniques
∗   Special circumstances

CLINICAL REASONING

1. Organize or cluster your findings for this patient by body system or concepts.

2. Analyze data collected. (Which data deviate from expected findings? Which additional data are needed?)

3. Using the analysis above, determine nursing diagnoses for this patient.

CHAPTER 21 Assessment of the Older Adult

With your lab partner assuming the role of the patient, conduct a focused history and examination. Your "student patient" may role-play a person with a particular symptom.

HISTORY

BIOGRAPHIC DATA

Date	Name			Gender M F
Date of birth	Age	Race	Marital status S M D W	Occupation

PRESENTING PROBLEM

History of Present Illness

Symptom Analysis of Presenting Problem (Onset, Location, Duration, Characteristics, Aggravating and Alleviating factors, Related symptoms, Treatment, Severity)

PRESENT HEALTH STATUS

Current health conditions:

Current medications: Prescription/Over-the-Counter/Herbal (Document if no medications are taken)

Name of Drug	Dosage/Frequency	Last Dose Taken	Reason for Taking

Allergies: Medication/Food/Other (Latex, contrast, iodine) (Document if there are no allergies)

Allergic To	Type of Reaction

Current Medical Treatments:

Treatment Modality	Reason for Treatment

PAST HEALTH HISTORY

List previous medical conditions, surgeries, hospitalizations, or injuries. (Document if none apply)

Name and Type	Date	Residual Problems

Immunizations: (date)

Varicella _____   Pneumococcal 13 _____   Pneumococcal 23 _____   Influenza _____   Tetanus _____

Date of Last Examinations

Physical examination:_____   Vision examination: _____

Hearing examination: _____   Dental examination: _____

FAMILY HISTORY (Indicate age and current health. If deceased, indicate age and cause of death.)

Person	Age	Current Health	Person	Age	Current Health
Mother			Father		
Sister			Brother		
Sister			Brother		
Daughter			Son		
Daughter			Son		

PERSONAL AND PSYCHOSOCIAL HISTORY (level of functioning, social, family interactions, and feelings about retirement)

Personal Status (feelings about fixed income, downsizing household, living alone, and other appropriate questions for patient's situation)

Family and Social Relationships (current living arrangements, access to friends and support systems, pets at home, involvement in family and friend activities, and any conflicts related to relationships)

Diet and Nutrition (typical diet and food preferences, allergies, tolerances, supplements, habits related to food or eating)

Functional Ability (patient's ability to perform self-care activities[†])

Dressing ❑   Toileting ❑   Bathing ❑   Eating ❑

Ambulating ❑   Shopping ❑   Cooking ❑   Housekeeping ❑

[†]If unable to perform independently, describe.

Mental Health (coping, loneliness, depression, anxiety, changes in memory)

Sleep (sleeping location, quality of sleep, hours per night, daytime naps, use of medications for sleep)

Tobacco, Alcohol, and Illicit Drug Use

Tobacco use: Y ❑ N ❑	Packs per day:
Alcohol intake: Y ❑ N ❑	Drinks per day:
Illicit drug use: Y ❑ N ❑	Describe:

Health Promotion Practices   Describe

Exercise (type/frequency):	
Stress management:	
Sleep habits:	
Self-examination (type/frequency):	
Use of seat belts:	
Other:	

Environment (safety, comfort, hazards in home and neighborhood)

Safety devices: (e.g., smoke alarms)	
Potential hazards:	
Within home	
Within neighborhood	

REVIEW OF SYSTEMS (Check all symptoms that apply, add comment below)

General Symptoms			
Pain ❑	Fatigue ❑	Weakness ❑	Fever ❑
Problems sleeping ❑	Unexplained changes in weight ❑		
Comments:			

Integumentary System			
Change in skin color/texture ❑	Frequent bruising ❑	Skin dryness or scaling ❑	Skin lesions ❑
Sores that do not heal ❑	Rashes ❑	Itching ❑	Change in nail texture ❑
Use of sunscreen ❑	Changes in hair texture ❑	Changes in hair distribution ❑	
Comments:			

Head			
Headaches ❑	Fainting ❑	Dizziness ❑	
Comments:			

Eyes			
Change in vision ❑	Difficulty reading ❑	Problems with night vision ❑	Dry or irritated eyes ❑
Wear corrective lenses ❑	If yes: How long?		
Comments:			

Ears			
Diminished hearing ❑	Hearing assistive device ❑	Ringing in ears ❑	Excessive earwax ❑
Comments:			

Nose and Mouth			
Dry mouth and nose ❑	Nasal discharge ❑	Bleeding gums ❑	Sneezing ❑
Dentures ❑	Trouble chewing ❑	Trouble swallowing ❑	Teeth (tooth loss, caries, pain) ❑
Teeth brushing and flossing routine ❑			
Comments:			

Neck			
Neck pain ❑	Neck stiffness ❑		
Comments:			

Breasts			
Pain ❑	Breast changes ❑	Lumps ❑	Unilateral enlargement ❑
Comments:			

Respiratory System			
Frequent colds ❑	Wheezing ❑	Coughing up blood ❑	Night sweats ❑
Exposure to smoke ❑	Frequent handwashing ❑	Influenza vaccine ❑	Smoking cessation ❑
Comments:			

Cardiovascular System			
Chest pain ❑	Palpitations ❑	Shortness of breath (dyspnea) ❑	Dyspnea during sleep ❑
Coldness to extremities ❑	Discoloration ❑	Varicose veins ❑	Leg pain with activity ❑
Paresthesia ❑	Edema ❑	Screening for hypertension, cholesterol ❑	Limit salt and fat intake ❑
Exercise (types/frequency):			
Comments:			

Gastrointestinal System			
Unusual pattern of bowel movements ❑	Constipation ❑	Nausea/vomiting ❑	Abdominal pain ❑
Dietary analysis ❑			
Comments:			

Urinary System			
Urgency ❑	Frequency ❑	Incontinence ❑	Nocturia ❑
Males			
Difficulty starting urine stream ❑	Weak urine stream ❑	Incomplete bladder emptying ❑	
Comments:			

Musculoskeletal System			
Muscle pain ❑	Muscle weakness ❑	Joint pain ❑	Stiffness ❑
Limitations in range of motion ❑	Change in mobility, gait, or balance ❑	Fall, injury history ❑	Use of assistive devices ❑
Amount and kind of exercise ❑	Osteoporosis screening ❑		
Comments:			

Neurologic System			
Headache ❑	Difficulty communicating ❑	Fainting ❑	Changes in movement ❑
Changes in sensation ❑	Changes in memory ❑	Problems with coordination ❑	Gait coordination ❑
Comments:			

Reproductive System			
Men			
Sexually active ❑	Impotence ❑		
Women			
Sexually active ❑	Vaginal dryness ❑	Vaginal itching ❑	Vaginal bleeding ❑
Comments:			

HEALTH PROMOTION AND PROTECTION

1. Identify risk factors for this patient.

2. Recommend health promotion activities for this patient.

EXAMINATION

The scope of examination techniques used with the older adult is the same as for the younger adult. The methods of evaluation and findings often differ. Guidelines for a basic examination are described below.

Examination Technique	Findings (document findings below)
► PERFORM hand hygiene.	
Vital Signs and Baseline Measurement ► MEASURE temperature, heart and respiratory rate, blood pressure.	*Vital Signs and Baseline Measurement* Temperature: Heart rate: Blood pressure: Respiratory rate:
► MEASURE height and weight.	Height: Weight:
► DETERMINE BMI.	BMI:

Examination Technique	Findings (document findings below)
▶ PERFORM hand hygiene.	
Vital Signs, Height, and Weight ▶ MEASURE temperature, blood pressure, pulse, and respirations. ▶ MEASURE height and weight. ▶ Determine BMI.	***Measurements*** Temperature: Heart rate: Blood pressure: Respiratory rate: Height: Weight: BMI:
Skin ▶ INSPECT the skin for color and lesions. ▶ PALPATE the skin for texture, temperature, moisture, turgor, and thickness.	***Skin***
Hair ▶ INSPECT and PALPATE the scalp and hair for surface characteristics, hair distribution, texture, quantity, and color. ▶ INSPECT facial and body hair for distribution, quantity, and texture.	***Hair***
Nails ▶ INSPECT and PALPATE the finger- and toenails for shape, contour, consistency, color, thickness, and cleanliness.	***Nails***

Examination Technique	Findings (document findings below)
Head ▶ INSPECT the head for shape, and skin characteristics. ▶ INSPECT facial structures for size, symmetry, movement, intactness, skin characteristics, and facial expressions. ✳ PALPATE the bony structures of the face and jaw for tenderness and jaw movement. ✳ PALPATE the temporal arteries for pulsations, texture, and tenderness.	*Head*
Vision ▶ TEST visual acuity (distant vision). ▶ TEST visual acuity (near vision). *Eye* ▶ INSPECT the external ocular structures. • Eyebrows, eyelashes, and eyelids for symmetry, skin characteristics, and discharge. • Conjunctiva for color, moisture, drainage, lesions. ▶ INSPECT the ocular structures. • Corneal light reflex for symmetry (Hirschberg's test). • Sclera for color and surface characteristics. • Cornea for transparency and surface characteristics. • Iris for shape and color. • Pupils for size, shape, reaction to light and accommodation, and consensual reaction.	*Eyes, Vision* Right eye, left eye, and both eyes

Examination Technique	Findings (document findings below)
▶ ASSESS visual fields for peripheral vision (Confrontation test). ✳ INSPECT the anterior chamber for transparency, iris surface, and chamber depth. ✳ INSPECT intraocular structures (ophthalmoscopic examination). • Inspect for a red reflex. • Inspect the optic disc for discrete margin, shape, size, color, and physiologic cup. • Inspect the retinal vessels for color, arteriolar light reflex, artery-to-vein ratio, and arteriovenous crossing changes. • Inspect the retinal background for color, presence of microaneurysms, hemorrhages, and exudates. • Inspect the macula for color and surface characteristics.	
Ear ▶ ASSESS hearing based on response from conversation. ▶ INSPECT the external ears. • Notice the alignment and position. • Inspect for size, symmetry, skin color, and skin intactness. • Inspect the external auditory meatus for discharge or lesions. ✳ INSPECT the internal ear structures. • Palpate the external ears and mastoid processes for characteristics, tenderness, and edema. • Inspect the external ear canal for cerumen, odor, edema, erythema, discharge, and foreign bodies. • Inspect the tympanic membrane for landmarks, color, contour, translucence, and fluctuation.	*Ears, Hearing*

Examination Technique	Findings (document findings below)

✳ TEST the acoustic cranial nerve to evaluate auditory function.
   • Whispered voice test
 	
   • Finger-rubbing test
 	
   • Weber's test
 	
   • Rinne test
 	
   • Audioscope	

Nose and Sinuses ▶ INSPECT the nose for appearance, symmetry, and discharge. ✳ PALPATE the nose for tenderness and ASSESS for patency. ✳ INSPECT internal nasal cavity for surface characteristics, lesions, erythema, discharge, and foreign bodies. ✳ PALPATE the frontal and maxillary paranasal sinuses for tenderness. ✳ TRANSILLUMINATE the sinus area for dim red glow.	***Nose and Sinuses***

Examination Technique	Findings (document findings below)

Mouth and Oropharynx
 	
▶ INSPECT the mouth and oropharynx.
   • Lips for color, symmetry, moisture, and texture.
 	
   • Teeth and gums for condition, color, surface characteristics, and alignment.
 	
   • Tongue for movement, color, and surface characteristics.
 	
   • Buccal mucosa and anterior and posterior pillars for color, surface characteristics, and odor.
 	
   • Palate, uvula, posterior pharynx, tonsils for texture, color, surface characteristics, and movement.
 	
✳ PALPATE the teeth, inner lip, and gums for condition and tenderness.
 	
✳ PALPATE the tongue for texture.
	Mouth and Oropharynx

Neck
 	
▶ INSPECT the neck.
   • Position in relation to the head and trachea.
 	
   • Skin characteristics, presence of lumps and masses.
 	
✳ ESTIMATE the range of motion of neck.
 	
✳ PALPATE the neck for anatomic structures and trachea.
 	
✳ PALPATE the thyroid gland for size, consistency, tenderness, and presence of nodules.
 	
✳ PALPATE lymph nodes for size, consistency, mobility, and tenderness.
	Neck
	
	Thyroid
	
	Lymph Nodes

Examination Technique	Findings (document findings below)
Lungs and Respiratory System ▶ INSPECT the patient for appearance, posture, and breathing effort. ▶ OBSERVE respirations for breathing pattern and chest expansion.	**Lungs and Respiratory System**
Posterior Thorax ▶ INSPECT the posterior thorax for shape, symmetry, and muscle development. ▶ AUSCULTATE the posterior and lateral thorax for breath sounds. ✳ PALPATE posterior thoracic muscles for tenderness and symmetry. ✳ PALPATE the posterior chest wall for thoracic expansion. ✳ PALPATE the posterior thoracic wall for vocal (tactile) fremitus.	**Posterior Thorax**
Anterior Thorax ▶ INSPECT the anterior thorax for shape and symmetry, muscle development, and costal angle. ▶ INSPECT anterior thorax for anteroposterior to lateral diameter. ▶ AUSCULTATE the anterior thorax for breath sounds. ✳ PALPATE the trachea for position. ✳ PALPATE the anterior thoracic muscles for tenderness and symmetry. ✳ PALPATE the anterior chest wall for thoracic expansion. ✳ PALPATE the anterior thoracic wall for vocal (tactile) fremitus.	**Anterior Thorax**

Examination Technique	Findings (document findings below)
Peripheral Vascular System ▶ PALPATE temporal and carotid pulses for amplitude. ▶ INSPECT the jugular vein for pulsations. ▶ INSPECT and PALPATE the upper extremities for symmetry and skin turgor. ▶ INSPECT and PALPATE the upper extremities for skin integrity, color, and temperature; capillary refill; and color and angle of nail beds. ▶ PALPATE brachial and radial pulses for rate, rhythm, amplitude, and contour. ▶ INSPECT and PALPATE the lower extremities for symmetry and skin turgor. ▶ INSPECT and PALPATE the lower extremities for skin integrity, color, temperature, hair distribution, capillary refill, color and angle of nail beds, superficial veins, and gross sensation. ▶ PALPATE the lower extremities for femoral, popliteal, posterior tibial pulses, and dorsalis pedis pulses for amplitude.	***Peripheral Vascular System***

Heart
 ▶ INSPECT the anterior chest wall for contour, pulsations, lifts, heaves, and retractions.
 	
 ▶ PALPATE the apical pulse for location.
 	
 ▶ AUSCULTATE S_1 and S_2 heart sounds for rate, rhythm, pitch, and splitting.
   • ASSESS heart rate.
 	
   • ASSESS rhythm.
 	
   • ASSESS pitch.
 	
   • ASSESS splitting.
 	
 ▶ Calculate the pulse deficit.
	Heart

Examination Technique	Findings (document findings below)
Peripheral Vascular System	*Peripheral Vascular System*
✳ AUSCULTATE the carotid artery for bruits.	
✳ PALPATE the epitrochlear lymph nodes.	
✳ PALPATE the inguinal lymph nodes.	
✳ MEASURE leg circumferences.	
✳ CALCULATE the ankle-brachial index.	
Abdominal and Gastrointestinal System	*Abdominal and Gastrointestinal System*
▶ INSPECT the abdomen for skin color, surface characteristics, venous patterns, contour, symmetry, and surface movements.	
▶ AUSCULTATE the abdomen for bowel sounds.	
▶ AUSCULTATE the abdomen for arterial and venous vascular sounds.	
▶ PALPATE the abdomen lightly for tenderness and muscle tone.	
▶ PALPATE the abdomen deeply for pain, masses, and pulsations.	

Examination Technique	Findings (document findings below)
✳ PERCUSS the abdomen for tones.	
✳ PERCUSS the liver to determine span and descent.	
✳ PERCUSS the spleen for size.	
✳ PALPATE the liver for lower border and pain.	
✳ PALPATE the gallbladder for pain.	
✳ PALPATE the spleen for border and tenderness.	
✳ PALPATE the kidneys for presence, contour, and tenderness.	
✳ PERCUSS the kidneys for costovertebral angle (CVA) tenderness.	
Musculoskeletal System ▶ INSPECT axial skeleton and extremities for alignment, symmetry, and gross deformities. ▶ INSPECT muscle groups for size and symmetry. ▶ PALPATE bones for pain; joints for pain, temperature, and edema; and muscles for pain, temperature, edema, and tone. ▶ OBSERVE range of motion for major joints and adjacent muscles, for pain on movement, joint stability, and deformity. ▶ TEST muscle strength and compare sides.	*Musculoskeletal System*

Examination Technique	Findings (document findings below)

Neurologic System
▶ ASSESS mental status and level of consciousness.
 	
▶ ASSESS speech for articulation and voice quality and comprehension of verbal communication.
 	
▶ NOTICE cranial nerve functions.
  • CN I (olfactory)—smell
 	
  • CN II (optic nerve)—ability to move in environment and see chair to sit
 	
  • CN III (oculomotor), IV (trochlear), VI (abducens)—eye movement
 	
  • CN V (trigeminal)—eye blink
 	
  • CN VII (facial)—face is symmetric during talking or smiling
 	
  • CN VIII (acoustic)—ability to hear
 	
  • CN IX (glossopharyngeal), CN X (vagus)—swallowing and ability to handle saliva
 	
  • CN X (vagus)—guttural speech sounds
 	
  • CN XI (spinal accessory)—shrug shoulders or turn head
 	
▶ OBSERVE gait for balance and symmetry.
 	
▶ EVALUATE extremities for muscle strength.
	Neurologic System

Examination Technique	Findings (document findings below)

Neurologic System
✳ ASSESS individual cranial nerves.
  • TEST nose for smell.
 	
  • TEST eyes for visual acuity.
 	
  • TEST eyes for peripheral vision.
 	
  • OBSERVE eyes for extraocular muscle movement.
 	
  • OBSERVE eyes for pupillary size, shape, equality, constriction, and accommodation.
 	
  • EVALUATE face for movement and sensation.
 	
  • TEST ears for hearing.
 	
  • TEST tongue for taste.
 	
  • INSPECT oropharynx for gag reflex and movement of soft palate.
 	
  • TEST tongue for movement, symmetry, strength, and absence of tumors.
 	
  • TEST shoulders and neck muscles for strength, movement, and symmetry.
 	
✳ TEST cerebellar function for balance and coordination. (Use at least two techniques.)
  • TEST for balance.
    • Romberg test
 	
    • With eyes closed, stand on one foot, then the other
 	
    • Heel-to-toe walking
 	
    • Hop on one foot, then the other
 	
    • Deep knee bends
 	
    • Walk on toes, then on heels	

Examination Technique	Findings (document findings below)

• EVALUATE upper extremity coordination.
   • Alternately tap hands to thighs
 	
   • With eyes closed and outstretched arms, touch finger to own nose
 	
   • Touch each finger to thumb in rapid sequence
 	
   • Rapidly move finger between nose and nurse's finger
 	
• EVALUATE lower extremity coordination.
   • Lying supine, slide heel down opposite shin
 	
✱ ASSESS sensory function.
   • ASSESS sensation to light touch.
 	
   • ASSESS sharp and dull sensation.
 	
   • ASSESS vibratory sense using tuning fork.
 	
   • ASSESS kinesthetic sensation or test of proprioception.
 	
   • TEST stereognosis.
 	
   • TEST two-point discrimination.
 	
   • TEST for extinction.
 	
   • EVALUATE graphesthesia.
 	
   • TEST point location.
 	
   • ASSESS peripheral sensation using a monofilament.	

Examination Technique	Findings (document findings below)

✻ EVALUATE extremities for deep tendon reflexes.
   • Triceps reflex
 	
   • Biceps reflex
 	
   • Brachioradial reflex
 	
   • Patellar reflex
 	
   • Achilles tendon
 	
✻ EVALUATE plantar reflex.
 	
✻ EVALUATE ankle clonus.	

Breasts *Female* ▶ INSPECT breasts for size, shape, contour, and symmetry. ▶ INSPECT the skin of the breasts for color, surface characteristics, and venous patterns. ▶ INSPECT the areolae for color, shape, and surface characteristics. ▶ INSPECT the nipples for position, symmetry, surface characteristics, lesions, bleeding, and discharge. ✻ INSPECT the breasts in various positions for bilateral pull, symmetry, and contour. ✻ INSPECT and PALPATE the axillae for enlarged lymph nodes, rash, lesions, or masses. ✻ PALPATE the breasts for tissue characteristics. ✻ PALPATE the nipples for surface characteristics and discharge.	**Breasts** *Female*

Examination Technique	Findings (document findings below)
Male ► INSPECT the breasts and nipples for symmetry, color, size, shape, rash, and lesions. ✳ PALPATE the breasts and nipples for surface characteristics, tenderness, size, and masses. ✳ PALPATE the axillae for lymph nodes.	*Male*
Female Reproductive ► Don examination gloves. ► INSPECT the pubic hair and skin over the mons pubis and inguinal area for distribution and surface characteristics. ► INSPECT and PALPATE the labia majora, labia minora, and clitoris for pigmentation and surface characteristics. ► INSPECT the urethral meatus, vaginal introitus, and perineum for positioning and surface characteristics. ► INSPECT and PALPATE the sacrococcygeal areas for surface characteristics and tenderness. ► INSPECT the perianal area and anus for color and surface characteristics. ✳ PALPATE the Skene and Bartholin glands for surface characteristics, discharge, and pain. ✳ PALPATE the vaginal wall for tone. ✳ PALPATE the rectal wall for muscle tone. ✳ ASSESS the anal sphincter for muscle tone. ✳ EXAMINE stool for characteristics and presence of occult blood.	*Female Reproductive*

Examination Technique	Findings (document findings below)
Male	*Male*
► PERFORM hand hygiene.	
► DON examination gloves.	
► INSPECT the pubic hair for distribution and skin for general characteristics.	
► INSPECT and PALPATE the penis for surface characteristics, color, tenderness, and discharge.	
► INSPECT the scrotum for color, texture, surface characteristics, and position.	
► INSPECT the inguinal region and the femoral area for bulges.	
► INSPECT and PALPATE the sacrococcygeal areas for surface characteristics and tenderness.	
► INSPECT the perianal area and anus for pigmentation and surface characteristics.	
✻ PALPATE the scrotum for surface characteristics and tenderness.	
✻ PALPATE the testes, epididymides, and vasa deferentia for location, consistency, tenderness, and nodules.	
✻ ASSESS the anal sphincter for tone.	
✻ PALPATE the anal canal and rectum for surface characteristics.	
✻ EXAMINE the stool for characteristics and presence of occult blood.	

► Routine techniques
✻ Special circumstances

CLINICAL REASONING

1. Organize or cluster your findings for this patient by body system or concepts.

2. Analyze data collected. (Which data deviate from expected findings? Which additional data are needed?)

3. Determine nursing diagnoses for this patient.

CHAPTER 22 Conducting a Head-to-Toe Examination

With your lab partner assuming the role of a patient, conduct a comprehensive history (Chapter 2) and examination (Chapter 22). Your "student patient" may role-play a person with a particular symptom.

BIOGRAPHIC DATA

Date	Name				Gender M F
Date of birth	Age	Race		Marital status S M D W	Occupation

During the history, perform a general survey for the following:

- OBSERVE the patient's appearance including hygiene and skin color.

- ASSESS level of consciousness and mental status.

- OBSERVE posture and mobility.

- ASSESS the patient's mood or affect.

- NOTICE the patient's ability to hear and speak.

- NOTICE the patient's breathing effort.

Reason for Seeking Care/Presenting Problem

History of Present Illness

Symptom Analysis of Presenting Problem (Onset, Location, Duration, Characteristics, Aggravating and Alleviating factors, Related symptoms, Treatment, Severity)

Present Health Status (current health conditions/chronic illnesses)

Current medications (prescription, over-the-counter, herbs, and vitamins): (Document if no medications are taken)

Name of Drug	Dosage/Frequency	Last Dose Taken	Reason for Taking

Current Medical Treatments (e.g., breathing treatments, dialysis, wound dressing): (Document if no medical treatments are used)

Allergies to Medication/Foods/Medical Products/Other (e.g., latex, contrast, tape): (Document if there are no allergies)

Allergic To	Type of Reaction

PAST HEALTH HISTORY

Childhood Illnesses (Check all that apply):

Measles ❑   Mumps ❑   Rubella ❑   Chickenpox ❑

Pertussis ❑   Influenza ❑   Ear infections ❑   Throat infections ❑

Other (describe) ❑

List previous medical conditions, surgeries, hospitalizations, or injuries. (Document if none apply)

Name and Type	Date	Residual Problems

Immunization	Date/s	Immunization	Date/s
Diphtheria, tetanus, acellular pertussis (DTaP)		*Haemophilus influenzae* type b (Hib)	
Hepatitis A		Hepatitis B	
Human papillomavirus (HPV)		Inactivated poliomyelitis (IPV)	
Influenza vaccine		Measles, mumps, rubella (MMR)	
Meningococcal conjugate vaccine (MCV)		Pneumococcal conjugate (PCV13)	
Pneumococcal polysaccharide (PPSV23)		Rotavirus	
Tetanus (Td)		Varicella	
Other		Other	

Last Examinations:

Last Examination	Date	Outcome
Last Physical		
Last Vision		
Last Dental		
Other (describe)		
Women Only		
Last Menstrual Period (LMP)		
Last Pregnancy		Gravida (number of pregnancies) _____ Para (number of births) _____ Abortion/miscarriage _____
Last Pap Smear		
Last Mammogram		

FAMILY HISTORY (Indicate age and current health. If deceased, indicate age and cause of death.)

Person	Age	Current Health	Person	Age	Current Health
Mother			Father		
Sister			Brother		
Sister			Brother		
Daughter			Son		
Daughter			Son		

Draw a genogram for your lab partner's family history.

PERSONAL AND PSYCHOSOCIAL HISTORY

Personal Status (feelings about self, cultural/religious affiliations and practices, education/work satisfaction, hobbies and interests)

Family and Social Relationships (significant others, individuals in home, role within family)

Diet/Nutrition (appetite, typical food and fluid intake, dietary restrictions, use of dietary supplements)

Functional Ability (patient's ability to perform self-care activities†)

Dressing ❑   Toileting ❑   Bathing ❑   Eating ❑

Ambulating ❑   Shopping ❑   Cooking ❑   Housekeeping ❑

†If unable to perform independently, describe.

Mental Health (anxiety, depression, irritability, stressful events, personal coping strategies)

Tobacco, Alcohol, and Illicit Drug Use

Tobacco use: Y ❑ N ❑	Packs per day:
Alcohol intake: Y ❑ N ❑	Drinks per day:
Illicit drug use: Y ❑ N ❑	Describe:

Health Promotion   **Describe**

Exercise (type/frequency):	
Stress management:	
Sleep habits:	
Self-examination (type/frequency):	
Use of seat belts:	
Oral hygiene practice (frequency of brushing/flossing):	
Other:	

Environment (include living and work environment)   **Describe**

Safety devices: (e.g., smoke alarms)	
Potential hazards:	
Within home	
Within neighborhood	

REVIEW OF SYSTEMS (Check all that apply and comment below; document if no symptoms reported.)

General Symptoms			
Pain ❏	Fatigue ❏	Weakness ❏	Fever ❏
Problems sleeping ❏	Unexplained changes in weight ❏		
Comments:			

Integumentary System			
Change in skin color/ texture ❏	Frequent bruising ❏	Itching ❏	Skin lesions ❏
Sores that do not heal ❏	Change in mole ❏	Change in amount, texture, or distribution of hair ❏	Change in texture of nails ❏
Rashes ❏	Excessive dryness ❏	Use of sunscreen? ❏	
Comments:			

Head			
Headaches ❏	Head injury ❏	Dizziness ❏	Fainting spells ❏
Use of protective headgear ❏			
Comments:			

Eyes			
Change in vision ❏	Discharge ❏	Excessive tearing ❏	Eye pain ❏
Sensitivity to light ❏	Flashing lights ❏	Halos around lights ❏	Difficulty reading ❏
Do you wear corrective lenses? ❏	If yes, how long? _____	Date last evaluated? _____	Use of protective eyewear ❏
Comments:			

Ears

Ear pain ❑	Drainage ❑	Recurrent infections ❑	Excessive earwax ❑
Changes in hearing ❑	Ringing in ears ❑	Sensitivity to noises ❑	Use of hearing device ❑
Protect ears from excessively loud noises ❑			
Comments:			

Nose, Nasopharynx, Sinuses

Nasal discharge ❑	Frequent nosebleeds ❑	Sneezing ❑	Nasal obstruction ❑
Sinus pain ❑	Postnasal drip ❑	Change in smell ❑	Snoring ❑
Comments:			

Mouth/Oropharynx

Sore throat ❑	Sore in mouth ❑	Bleeding gums ❑	Change in taste ❑
Trouble chewing ❑	Trouble swallowing ❑	Dental prosthesis ❑	Change in voice ❑
Teeth brushing and flossing routine ❑			
Comments:			

Neck

Lymph node enlargement ❑	Swelling or mass in neck ❑	Neck pain ❑	Neck stiffness ❑
Comments:			

Breasts

Pain ❑	Swelling ❑	Lumps or masses ❑	Change in appearance ❑
Nipple discharge ❑	Do you perform breast self-examinations? ❑	If yes, how often? _____	
Comments:			

Respiratory System

Frequent colds ❑	Shortness of breath (dyspnea) ❑	Wheezing ❑	Pain with breathing ❑
Cough ❑	Coughing up blood ❑	Night sweats ❑	Exposure to smoke ❑
Frequent handwashing ❑	Influenza vaccine ❑	Smoking cessation ❑	
Comments:			

Cardiovascular System

Chest pain ❑	Palpitations ❑	Shortness of breath (dyspnea) ❑	Dyspnea during sleep ❑
Cold extremities ❑	Discoloration ❑	Varicose veins ❑	Leg pain with activity ❑
Paresthesia ❑	Edema ❑	Screening for hypertension ❑	Screening for cholesterol ❑
Limit salt and fat intake ❑	Exercise (types/frequency):		
Comments:			

Gastrointestinal System

Pain ❑	Heartburn ❑	Nausea/vomiting ❑	Vomiting blood ❑
Jaundice ❑	Change in appetite ❑	Diarrhea ❑	Constipation ❑
Change in bowel habits ❑	Blood in stools ❑	Hemorrhoids ❑	Dietary analysis ❑
Colon cancer screening ❑			
Comments:			

Urinary System

Hesitancy ❑	Frequency ❑	Urgency ❑	Nocturia ❑
Pain with urination ❑	Flank pain ❑	Blood in urine ❑	Excessive urinary volume ❑
Decreased urinary volume ❑	Change in stream ❑	Flank pain ❑	Incontinence ❑
Comments:			

Reproductive System				
	Lesions ❑	Discharge ❑	Pain or masses ❑	
Females:	Pain during menses ❑	Heavy or prolonged menses ❑	No menses ❑	
Are you currently involved in a sexual relationship(s)?	Y ❑ N ❑	If yes, what is the nature of the relationship(s) (heterosexual, homosexual, bisexual)?		
Number of sexual partners in last 3 months?				
Do you protect yourself from sexually transmitted diseases (STDs)?	Y ❑ N ❑	If yes, method(s) used:		
Do you use birth control?	Y ❑ N ❑	If yes, method(s) used:		
Problems with sexual activity				
Painful intercourse ❑	Change in sex drive ❑	Infertility ❑	Impotence ❑	
Comments:				

Musculoskeletal System			
Muscle pain ❑	Muscle weakness ❑	Joint swelling ❑	Joint pain ❑
Joint stiffness ❑	Limitations in range of motion ❑	Limitations in mobility ❑	Back pain ❑
Use of body mechanics ❑	Osteoporosis screening ❑		
Comments:			

Neurologic System			
Pain ❑	Seizures ❑	Fainting ❑	Changes in cognition ❑
Changes in memory ❑	Problems with coordination ❑	Tremor ❑	Spasms ❑
Changes in sensation ❑	Disorientation ❑		
Comments:			

HEALTH PROMOTION AND PROTECTION

1. Identify risk factors for this patient.

2. Recommend health promotion activities for this patient.

EXAMINATION

Examination Technique	Findings (document findings below)
Routine Techniques (except where indicated)	
▶ PERFORM hand hygiene.	
Vital Signs and Baseline Measurement ▶ MEASURE vital signs.	***Vital Signs and Baseline Measurement*** Temperature: Heart rate: Blood pressure: Respiratory rate:
▶ MEASURE height and weight.	Height: Weight:
▶ DETERMINE BMI.	BMI:
▶ ASSESS visual acuity.	Visual acuity: Left eye: Right eye: Both eyes:

Examination Technique	Findings (document findings below)
Examine Hands with Patient Seated ▶ INSPECT skin surface characteristics, temperature, and moisture. ▶ INSPECT for symmetry. ▶ INSPECT and PALPATE nails for shape, contour, consistency, color, thickness, and cleanliness. ▶ OBSERVE for clubbing of fingers. ▶ TEST capillary refill.	***Examine Hands with Patient Seated***
Examine Head and Face ▶ INSPECT the head for size, shape, and position. ▶ INSPECT the skin and scalp for characteristics. If indicated: • palpate structures of the skull for contour, symmetry, tenderness, and intactness. • palpate scalp for tenderness and intactness. • palpate temporal pulses for pulsation, amplitude, and tenderness.	***Examine Head and Face***

Examination Technique	Findings (document findings below)
▶ INSPECT for facial structures for size, symmetry, movement, skin characteristics, and facial expression. If indicated: • palpate the structures of the skull for contour, symmetry, tenderness, and intactness. • palpate the bony structures of the face and jaw for tenderness and jaw movement. • ask patient to clench eyes tightly; wrinkle forehead; smile; stick out tongue; and puff out cheeks, noting symmetry. • evaluate sensation of forehead, cheeks, and chin to light touch. ▶ INSPECT skin for color and lesions. If indicated: • palpate skin for texture, tenderness, and lesions. • palpate facial bones for size, intactness, and tenderness.	

Examination Technique	Findings (document findings below)
Examine Eyes ► ASSESS peripheral vision. ► INSPECT eyebrows for skin characteristics and symmetry. ► INSPECT eyelids and eyelashes for symmetry, position, closure, blinking, and color. ► INSPECT conjunctiva and sclera for color and clarity; inspect cornea for transparency. If indicated: • inspect anterior chamber for transparency and chamber depth. • palpate the eye, eyelids, and lacrimal puncta for firmness, tenderness, and discharge. ► INSPECT symmetry of eye movements. If indicated: • test extraocular eye movements in six cardinal fields of gaze. • perform cover-uncover test.	***Examine Eyes***

Examination Technique	Findings (document findings below)
▶ INSPECT iris for shape and color.	
▶ EXAMINE the pupillary response, consensual reaction, corneal light reflex, and accommodation. If indicated: • inspect the anterior chamber for transparency and chamber depth. • perform ophthalmic examination: inspect red reflex, disc cup margins, vessels, retinal surface, and macula.	
Examine Ears ▶ INSPECT external ear for alignment, position, size, shape, symmetry, intactness, skin color, and presence of deformities. ▶ INSPECT external auditory canal for discharge or lesions. ▶ PALPATE lymph nodes of the head for size and tenderness. ▶ PALPATE external ear and mastoid areas for tenderness, edema, or nodules. If indicated: • perform whisper test to evaluate gross hearing. • perform Rinne and Weber tests for conduction and sensorineural losses. • perform otoscopic examination: inspect characteristics of external canal, cerumen, and eardrum (landmarks).	*Examine Ears*

Examination Technique	Findings (document findings below)
Examine Nose ▶ INSPECT nasal structure and septum for symmetry. ▶ INSPECT nose for patency, color of turbinates, and discharge. If indicated: • evaluate sense of smell. • palpate nose for tenderness and to assess for patency. • inspect internal nasal cavity for surface characteristics, lesions, erythema, discharge, and foreign bodies. • palpate the frontal and maxillary paranasal sinuses for tenderness. • transilluminate sinuses for dim red glow.	*Examine Nose*

Examination Technique	Findings (document findings below)
Examine Mouth ▶ INSPECT lips for color, symmetry, moisture, and texture. ▶ INSPECT teeth and gums for condition, color, surface characteristics, and alignment. ▶ INSPECT tongue for movement, symmetry, color, and surface characteristics. ▶ INSPECT buccal mucosa and anterior and posterior pillars for color, surface characteristics, and odor. ▶ INSPECT the palate, uvula, posterior pharynx, and tonsils for texture, color, surface characteristics, and movement. If indicated: • palpate teeth, inner lips, and gums for condition and tenderness with gloved hands. • palpate tongue for texture with gloved hands. • evaluate gag reflex. • test temporomandibular joint for movement.	*Examine Mouth*

Examination Technique	Findings (document findings below)
Examine Neck ▸ INSPECT the neck position in relation to the head and trachea. ▸ INSPECT the neck for skin characteristics and presence of lumps and masses. If indicated: • estimate range of motion. • palpate the neck for anatomic structures and trachea. • palpate the thyroid gland for size, consistency, tenderness, and presence of nodules. • palpate regional lymph nodes for size, consistency, mobility, and tenderness. • palpate the neck for tenderness and muscle strength. • test range of motion of head and neck • shrug shoulders against resistance.	*Examine Neck*
▸ PALPATE carotid pulses, one at a time, for amplitude. If indicated: • auscultate carotid arteries for bruits.	

Examination Technique	Findings (document findings below)
Examine Upper Extremities	*Examine Upper Extremities*
► INSPECT patient's arms for skin characteristics, symmetry, and color.	
► INSPECT the shoulders and shoulder girdle for equality of height, symmetry, and contour.	
► INSPECT the joints of the wrists and hands for symmetry, alignment, and number of digits.	
► PALPATE the shoulders for firmness, fullness, symmetry, and pain.	
► PALPATE the skin for texture, moisture, mobility, turgor, and thickness.	
► PALPATE the arms for temperature.	
► PALPATE elbows, wrists, and fingers for tenderness and deformities.	

Examination Technique	Findings (document findings below)
▶ PALPATE brachial or radial pulse for presence and amplitude. If indicated: • palpate epitrochlear lymph nodes for size, consistency, mobility, tenderness, and warmth. • palpate ulnar pulse for presence and amplitude. ▶ OBSERVE range of motion of shoulders, elbow, wrists, and fingers, ASSESS muscle strength of upper and lower arms. If indicated: • test deep tendon reflexes. • test for sensation of upper and lower arms.	
Assess Posterior Chest ▶ OBSERVE posterior and lateral chest for shape, muscular development, scapular placement, spine alignment, and posture. ▶ INSPECT skin for color, intactness, lesions, and scars. ▶ PALPATE vertebrae for alignment and tenderness.	*Assess Posterior Chest*

Examination Technique	Findings (document findings below)
▶ OBSERVE respiratory movement for symmetry, depth, and rhythm of respirations. If indicated: • palpate posterior thorax and muscles for tenderness and symmetry. • palpate posterior thorax for expansion. • palpate posterior thorax for fremitus. ▶ AUSCULTATE posterior and lateral thoraces for breath sounds.	
Assess Anterior Chest ▶ INSPECT skin for color, intactness, lesions, and scars. ▶ INSPECT anterior thorax for contour, pulsations, lift, heaves, and retractions. ▶ OBSERVE respiratory movement for symmetry, breathing pattern, and posture. ▶ INSPECT the anterior thorax for shape symmetry, muscle development, and costal angle. ▶ INSPECT anterior thorax for the anteroposterior to lateral diameter.	*Assess Anterior Chest*

Examination Technique	Findings (document findings below)
If indicated: • observe precordium for pulsations or heaving. • palpate the anterior thorax and muscles for tenderness and symmetry. • palpate anterior thoracic walls for expansion. • palpate anterior thoracic wall for fremitus. ▶ PALPATE left anterior thorax to locate point of maximum impulse (PMI). ▶ AUSCULTATE anterior thorax for breath sounds. ▶ AUSCULTATE heart for rate, rhythm, intensity, frequency, timing, and splitting of S_1 or S_2 or presence of S_3, S_4, or murmurs.	
Assess Breasts *Female Breasts* ▶ INSPECT for size, symmetry, shape, surface characteristics, and venous patterns. ▶ INSPECT areolae for color, shape, and surface characteristics.	***Assess Breasts*** *Female Breasts*

Examination Technique	Findings (document findings below)
▶ INSPECT nipples for position, symmetry, surface characteristics, lesions, bleeding, and discharge. If indicated: • inspect breasts in various positions for bilateral pull, symmetry, and contour.	
Male Breasts ▶ INSPECT the breasts and nipples for symmetry, color, size, shape, rashes, and lesions. ▶ PALPATE the breasts and nipples for surface characteristics, tenderness, size, and masses.	*Male Breasts*
All Patients If indicated: • inspect and palpate the axillae for enlarged lymph nodes, rashes, lesions, or masses.	*All Patients*
Assess Anterior Chest with Patient in Recumbent Position ▶ INSPECT for jugular vein pulsations. If indicated: • measure blood pressure with patient lying to compare with earlier reading.	***Assess Anterior Chest with Patient in Recumbent Position***

Examination Technique	Findings (document findings below)
Assess Female Breasts ▶ PALPATE breasts for tissue characteristics. ▶ PALPATE nipples for surface characteristics and discharge.	**Assess Female Breasts**
Assess Abdomen ▶ INSPECT the abdomen for skin color, surface characteristics, venous patterns, and contour. ▶ AUSCULTATE the abdomen for bowel sounds and arterial and venous sounds. ▶ PALPATE lightly all quadrants for tenderness and muscle tone. ▶ PALPATE deeply all quadrants for pain, masses, and aortic pulsations. If indicated: • percuss the abdomen for tones. • percuss the liver to determine span and descent. • percuss the spleen for size. • palpate the liver for lower border and pain.	**Assess Abdomen**

Examination Technique	Findings (document findings below)
• palpate the gallbladder for pain.	
• palpate the spleen for border and pain.	
• palpate the kidneys for contour and pain.	
• percuss the kidneys for costovertebral angle pain.	
▶ Patient raises head to evaluate flexion and strength of abdominal muscles and inspect for umbilical hernia.	
If indicated: • lightly palpate inguinal region for femoral pulses and bulges that may be associated with hernia.	
• palpate inguinal lymph nodes for size, consistency, mobility, tenderness, and warmth.	
Assess Lower Extremities ▶ INSPECT legs, ankles, and feet for symmetry, skin characteristics, vascular sufficiency, hair distribution, number of digits, and deformities. ▶ PALPATE lower legs for temperature.	***Assess Lower Extremities***

Examination Technique	Findings (document findings below)
▶ PALPATE lower legs, knees, ankles, and feet for tenderness and deformities.	
▶ PALPATE the dorsalis pedis pulses for presence and amplitude.	
▶ TEST capillary refill of toes.	
If indicated: • palpate popliteal and posterior tibial pulses.	
• calculate the ankle-brachial index.	
• measure circumference of each thigh and calf.	
▶ OBSERVE range of motion of hips, knees, ankles, and feet.	
▶ TEST motor strength of upper and lower legs.	
If indicated: • test for deep tendon reflexes and ankle clonus.	
• test sensation of hips, legs, ankles, and feet.	
• test for nerve root compression with straight leg raises.	

Examination Technique	Findings (document findings below)
Assess Remaining Neurologic and Musculoskeletal Systems ▶ OBSERVE patient moving from lying to sitting position; note use of muscles, ease of movement, and coordination. ▶ ASSESS patient's gait: observe and palpate patient's spine and posterior thorax for alignment as patient stands and bends forward to touch toes. ▶ INSPECT hips for symmetry. ▶ PALPATE the hips for stability and pain. If indicated: • evaluate hyperextension, lateral bending, and rotation of upper trunk. • test sensory function by using light and deep sensation. • test and compare vibratory sensation bilaterally. • test proprioception. • test two-point discrimination. • test stereognosis and graphesthesia.	*Assess Remaining Neurologic and Musculoskeletal Systems*

Examination Technique	Findings (document findings below)
• test fine motor functioning and coordination of upper extremities.	
• test fine motor functioning and coordination of lower extremities.	
• evaluate Babinski sign.	
• assess cerebellar and motor function.	
Examine Genitalia, Pelvic Region, and Rectum: Males ► Patient is lying and adequately draped. Don examination gloves. ► INSPECT pubic hair for distribution and skin for general characteristics. ► INSPECT and PALPATE the penis for surface characteristics, color, tenderness, and discharge. ► INSPECT scrotum for color, texture, surface characteristics, and position. If indicated: • palpate the scrotum for surface characteristics and tenderness.	*Examine Genitalia, Pelvic Region, and Rectum: Males*

Examination Technique	Findings (document findings below)
▶ Position patient lying on left side with right hip and knee flexed.	
▶ INSPECT and PALPATE the sacrococcygeal areas for surface characteristics and tenderness.	
▶ INSPECT the perianal area and anus for pigmentation and surface characteristics. If indicated: • palpate anal canal and rectum for surface characteristics with lubricated gloved finger. • examine stool for characteristics and presence of occult blood. • palpate anus for sphincter tone. • palpate the anal canal and rectum for surface characteristics.	
Patient is standing. ▶ INSPECT inguinal region and femoral area for bulges.	

Examination Technique	Findings (document findings below)
If indicated: • palpate the testes, epididymides, and vasa deferentia for location, consistency, tenderness, and nodules. • palpate inguinal canal for hernias.	
Examine Genitalia, Pelvic Region, and Rectum: Females ▶ Patient should be lying in lithotomy position; the nurse should don examination gloves. ▶ INSPECT the pubic hair and skin for distribution and surface characteristics. ▶ INSPECT and PALPATE the labia majora, labia minora, and clitoris for pigmentation and surface characteristics. ▶ INSPECT the urethral meatus, vaginal introitus, and perineum for positioning and surface characteristics. ▶ INSPECT and PALPATE the sacrococcygeal areas for surface characteristics and tenderness. If indicated: • palpate the Skene and Bartholin glands for surface characteristics, discharge, and pain. • palpate vaginal wall for tone.	***Examine Genitalia, Pelvic Region, and Rectum: Females***

Examination Technique	Findings (document findings below)
▶ INSPECT the perianal area and anus for color and surface characteristics. If indicated: • palpate the rectal wall for surface characteristics. • assess the anal sphincter for muscle tone. • examine stool for characteristics and presence of occult blood when lubricated gloved finger removed. ▶ Patient resumes a seated position.	

CLINICAL REASONING

1. Organize or cluster your findings for this patient by body system or concepts.

2. Analyze data collected. (Which data deviate from expected findings? Which additional data are needed?)

3. Determine nursing diagnoses for this patient.

CHAPTER 23 Documenting the Head-to-Toe Health Assessment

No laboratory activities are required for the content in this chapter.

CHAPTER **24** Adapting Health Assessment to the Hospitalized Patient

Practice what you learned by describing data you would collect for a focused assessment on hospitalized patients. Use the guidelines in Chapter 22 to help you organize your data collection. Below is an outline of a focused assessment.

OUTLINE

- Vital signs: Temperature, pulse, respirations, blood pressure, and oxygen saturation
- Orientation: To person, place, time, and situation
- Communication: Speech clear and appropriate
- Pain: Use OLD CARTS mnemonic to assess pain
- Skin: Turgor and intactness. *Assess any intravenous catheter sites, incisions, or wounds. Complete risk assessment for pressure ulcers. Assess extremities for edema.*
- Head, eyes, ears, nose, and throat: *Assess intactness and color of skin of nares if patient has a nasogastric tube or nasal prongs are providing oxygen. Assess intactness and color of skin of ears if nasal prongs or face mask is providing oxygen. Assess color of skin of face if face mask is providing oxygen. Assess drainage from nasogastric tube for color.*
- Cardiac and peripheral vascular system: S_1 and S_2, rate, rhythm; radial and pedal pulse rhythm and amplitude; warmth of extremities; capillary refill
- Lungs and respiratory system: Ease of breathing, skin color, symmetry of thorax, lung sounds
- Abdomen and gastrointestinal system: Appearance of abdomen, bowel sounds, light and deep palpation of the abdomen. *Assess colostomy or ileostomy for drainage and security of bag. Ensure indwelling urinary catheter is secured as needed; notice the coil of tubing and color of urine in tubing.*
- Musculoskeletal system: Compare right and left extremities for symmetry and muscle strength
- Neurologic system: Movement and sensation of extremities

EXAMPLE

Below is an example of data collected during a focused physical assessment of a patient. Move from head to toe. There are a variety of sequences that could be used. Be sure you are systematic and thorough. Include assessment of any equipment.

EXAMPLE: A patient had an open reduction with internal fixation of the left femur yesterday. She has a peripheral IV line in her left lower arm with 5% dextrose with normal saline (D_5NS) infusing at a rate of 100 mL/hr and a urinary catheter to bedside drainage. There is a sequential compression device (SCD) on her right leg. She is awake and alert. See Figures 24-3, 24-18, and 24-22.

Perform hand hygiene and clean the diaphragm and bell of your stethoscope.

With the patient in supine position,

- OBSERVE the patient's orientation to person, time, place, and situation.
- ASSESS speech for clarity and appropriateness.
- ASSESS pain using OLD CARTS mnemonic.
- INSPECT the patient for skin color and posture/position.

- OBSERVE the breathing pattern and chest expansion.
- COUNT respirations for rate.
- MEASURE the oxygen saturation.
- MEASURE the blood pressure in the right arm.
- MEASURE the oral temperature.
- PALPATE skin for turgor.
- PALPATE a radial pulse for rate and amplitude.
- INSPECT the IV site for redness, edema, and warmth. Verify correct IV fluid at the correct rate of flow.
- AUSCULTATE anterior and lateral thoraces for breath sounds; AUSCULTATE heart sounds for rhythm; INSPECT the skin of the abdomen for color, surface characteristics, and venous patterns. AUSCULTATE abdomen for bowel sounds. *[Note: complete all auscultation at once since your stethoscope is in hand.]*
- PALPATE all quadrants of the abdomen for tenderness and guarding.
- INSPECT the incision site for redness, edema, drainage, and pain.

Remove SCD from right leg.
- INSPECT legs, ankles, and feet for skin characteristics, vascular insufficiency, hair distribution, and deformities.
- PALPATE the legs for temperature. ASSESS capillary refill of toes bilaterally.
- PALPATE dorsalis pedis pulses bilaterally for presence and amplitude.
- ASSESS movement and sensation of toes bilaterally.
- ASSESS muscles of legs for strength.
- INSPECT the urine in the drainage tubing and bedside bag for color and sediment. ENSURE the tubing is free from kinks and the catheter is secured to the patient's inner thigh as needed.

Assist the patient to turn to her left side while you:
- AUSCULTATE the posterior thorax for breath sounds.
- INSPECT the skin on the buttocks for redness. PALPATE the skin for blanching.

Assist the patient to a comfortable position.

SAMPLE CASES

Below are brief summaries of three hospitalized patients. What data would you collect for a focused assessment of each one?

Patient A had abdominal surgery to repair a small bowel obstruction. His wound dehisced, requiring an abdominal dressing. He has a peripheral IV line in his right lower arm infusing 5% dextrose in normal saline (D_5NS) at a rate of 125 mL/hr. He has a nasogastric tube in his right naris attached to low intermittent suction. See Figures 24-3, 24-7, and 24-14.

Describe the data you would collect during a focused physical assessment of this patient, and include assessment of any equipment. Move from head to toe.

Perform hand hygiene and clean the diaphragm and bell of your stethoscope.

Patient B has a gastrostomy tube with bolus tube feedings every 6 hours followed by 250 mL of water. She has a saline well in her left arm used for medication administration only. She is receiving oxygen by nasal cannula at 3 liters per minute (LPM). See Figures 24-3, 24-8, 24-12, and 24-13.

Describe the data you would collect during a focused physical assessment of this patient, and include assessment of any equipment. Move from head to toe.

Perform hand hygiene and clean the diaphragm and bell of your stethoscope.

Patient C had a colectomy with a colostomy 2 days ago. She has a peripheral IV in her left lower arm infusing lactated Ringer's at a rate of 75 mL/hr. She has a wound drain with a bulb-type container to collect the drainage. She has a urinary catheter to bedside drainage. See Figures 24-3, 24-15, 24-16, 24-17, and 24-18.

Describe below the data you would collect during a focused physical assessment of this patient, and include assessment of any equipment. Move from head to toe.

Perform hand hygiene and clean the diaphragm and bell of your stethoscope.

Notes

Notes

Notes